The American Holistic Health
Association Complete Guide to

ALTERNATIVE
MEDICINE

The American Holistic Health Association Complete Guide to

ALTERNATIVE MEDICINE

WILLIAM COLLINGE, M.P.H., PH.D.

INTRODUCTION BY
LEN DUHL, M.D.
PROFESSOR, SCHOOL OF PUBLIC HEALTH
UNIVERSITY OF CALIFORNIA AT BERKELEY

WARNER BOOKS

A Time Warner Company

Warner Books, Inc., 1271 Avenue of the Americas, New York, NY 10020
W A Time Warner Company

Printed in the United States of America
First printing: January 1996
10 9 8 7 6 5 4 3 2

Library of Congress Cataloging-in-Publication Data

Collinge, William.
    [Complete guide to alternative medicine]
    The American Holistic Health Association Complete guide to
alternative medicine / William Collinge.
        p.   cm.
    Includes bibliographical references and index.
    ISBN 0-446-51817-4
    1. Alternative medicine.   I. American Holistic Health
Association.   II. Title.
    R733.C65   1996
    615.5—dc20   95-10201
                                                                       CIP

Book design by Giorgetta Bell McRee

To Rosie

Note to the Reader

Contents

A Message from the American Holistic
Health Association xi
Acknowledgments xiii
Introduction by Len Duhl, M.D. xvii
CHAPTER   1. THE CRISIS OF FREEDOM: HOW DO WE
                  CHOOSE? 1
CHAPTER   2. CHINESE MEDICINE: THE COSMIC
                  SYMPHONY... 13
CHAPTER   3. AYURVEDA: THE WISDOM
                  OF THE ANCIENTS... 55
CHAPTER   4. NATUROPATHIC MEDICINE: THE GREAT
                  CORNUCOPIA.. 96
CHAPTER   5. HOMEOPATHY: THE GRAND
                  PROVOCATEUR.. 134

CONTENTS

CHAPTER 6. MIND/BODY MEDICINE: THE DANCE OF
SOMA AND PSYCHE.................................... 167

CHAPTER 7. OSTEOPATHIC MEDICINE: STRUCTURE
AND FUNCTION AS ONE 205

CHAPTER 8. CHIROPRACTIC: OPENING THE GATES 232

CHAPTER 9. MASSAGE THERAPY AND BODYWORK:
HEALING THROUGH TOUCH 266

CHAPTER 10. NEW CHOICES, NEW REALITIES 307

Notes... 323

Index 349

About the Author 361

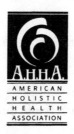

AMERICAN
HOLISTIC
HEALTH
ASSOCIATION

A Message from
the American Holistic Health Association

Creating wellness is an ongoing process. This book can help you take an important step toward wellness by becoming more informed about the many options available in the health care marketplace today. We encourage you to explore the traditions and therapies that feel appropriate for you and your situation.

Wherever you are on the path to achieving wellness, the American Holistic Health Association (AHHA) would like to support you. AHHA (pronounced *ah-ha*) is a nonprofit 501(C)(3) educational organization incorporated in 1989. Our goal is to promote health and well-being through personal responsibility, considering the whole person (physical, emotional, mental, spiritual), wellness-oriented lifestyle choices, and active participation in personal health decisions and healing.

To support you AHHA serves as a national clearinghouse

for information about conventional and complementary health resources. We provide a variety of educational materials including:

Educational Booklets for use in personal growth and development as well as health education programs that promote a wellness perspective.

Resource Lists of professional referral organizations, information research services for specific diseases and chronic conditions, catalogs of self-help tools and educational opportunities.

Award-winning Newsletter, *AhHa!,* to provide practical self-help suggestions, plus news about recent developments and research findings in the health and wellness field.

These resources are available to the public at no charge, thanks to contributions from our individual and organizational members.

Join the vital movement toward wellness. Bring greater quality of life to yourself and those you love. Call or write to request free materials or membership information:

AHHA—Dept C
P.O. Box 17400
Anaheim, CA 92817-7400
(714) 779-6152

Suzan V. Walter, President
American Holistic Health Association

Acknowledgments

Many people contributed to the fruition of this project. I particularly wish to thank my mentor in the School of Public Health at U.C. Berkeley, Len Duhl, M.D., grandfather of the Healthy Cities movement, whose course on alternative paradigms of health was a great source of inspiration. I also thank Suzan Walter and the board of the American Holistic Health Association for believing in this project; Joann Davis, my editor at Warner Books; Candice Fuhrman, my literary agent; and Annabel Gregory for her insight and support in the preparation of the manuscript.

The following people from the alternative medical traditions provided invaluable consultation and support. To each of them I extend my gratitude and deep respect for their work:

Joseph Helms, M.D., President, American Academy of Medical Acupuncture, and coordinator of physician education in acupuncture at UCLA Medical School

Daniel Kenner, O.M.D., L.Ac., private practice, Santa Rosa, CA

David Walker, O.M.D., L.Ac., private practice, Santa Rosa, CA

Nancy Carroll, L.Ac., private practice, Sebastopol, CA

Harriet Beinfield, L.Ac., and Efrem Korngold, O.M.D., L.Ac., Chinese Medicine Works, San Francisco, CA

Deepak Chopra, M.D., Director of the Center for Mind/Body Medicine, La Jolla, CA

Vivek Shanbhag, M.D., Head of the Department of Ayurvedic Medicine, Bastyr University of Natural Health Sciences, Seattle

Janhavi Morton, ayurveda practitioner, Santa Rosa, CA

Mary Jo Cravatta, D.C., private practice, Palo Alto, CA

Stuart Rothenberg, M.D., Dean, College of Maharishi Ayur-Ved, Maharishi International University, Fairfield, IA

Michael Murray, N.D., Bastyr University of Natural Health Sciences, Seattle, WA

Leanna Standish, N.D., Ph.D., Bastyr University of Natural Health Sciences, Seattle, WA

Jared Zeff, N.D., L.Ac., Academic Dean, National College of Naturopathic Medicine, Portland, OR

David Field, N.D., L.Ac., private practice, Santa Rosa, CA

Michael Carlston, M.D., D.Ht., University of California San Francisco Medical School, and Hahnemann Homeopathic Medical College, Albany, CA

Dana Ullman, M.P.H., President, Foundation for Homeopathic Education and Research, Berkeley, CA

Frederick Bishop, Executive Director, International Foundation for Homeopathy, Seattle, WA

Roger Morrison, M.D., and Nancy Herrick, P.A., Hahnemann Medical Clinic, Albany, CA

Durr Elmore, N.D., President, Homeopathic Association of Naturopathic Physicians, Mulino, OR

Claire Green, N.D., private practice, Santa Rosa, CA

Acknowledgments

Herbert Benson, M.D., President, Mind/Body Medical Institute, Harvard Medical School and New England Deaconess Hospital, Boston, MA

Cynthia Medich, Ph.D., R.N., Mind/Body Medical Institute, Harvard Medical School and New England Deaconess Hospital, Boston, MA

Lydia Temoshok, Ph.D., Global Program on AIDS, World Health Organization, Geneva, Switzerland

John Pammer, D.C., President, American Chiropractic Association, Arlington, VA

William Meeker, D.C., President, Consortium for Chiropractic Research and Dean of Research, Palmer College of Chiropractic-West, San Jose, CA

Donald Epstein, D.C., Founder, Network Chiropractic, Longmont, CA

Lawrence Oberstein, D.C., private practice, Santa Rosa, CA

Robert Dubin, D.C., private practice, Petaluma, CA

James Adams, D.C., private practice, Sonoma, CA

Terry Rondberg, D.C., President, World Chiropractic Alliance, Chandler, AZ

William Anderson, D.O., President, American Osteopathic Association, Chicago, IL

Carlisle Holland, D.O., Santa Rosa Medical Group, Santa Rosa, CA

Sister Anne Brooks, D.O., Tutwiler Clinic, Tutwiler, MS

Yusuf Erskine, D.O., private practice, Sebastopol, CA

Elliot Greene, M.A., President, American Massage Therapy Association, Evanston, IL

John Upledger, D.O., Founder, The Upledger Institute, Palm Beach Gardens, FL

James Schuelke, Executive Director, Rolf Institute, Boulder, CO

Bridget Beck, Certified Rolfer, private practice, Santa Rosa, CA

Rome Roberts Earle, Certified Teacher of the Alexander Technique, private practice, Oakland, CA

Tiffany Field, Ph.D., Director, Touch Research Institute, University of Miami Medical School, Miami, FL

Acknowledgments

Iona Marsaa Teeguarden, M.A., Founder and Director, Jin Shin Do® Foundation for Bodymind Acupressure™, Felton, CA

Joanna Cieppa, C.M.T., private practice, Sonoma County, CA

Gail Beth Gardener, Certified Rosen Practitioner, Sebastopol, CA

William Flocco, Director, American Academy of Reflexology, Burbank, CA

Craig Carr, L.Ac., Certified Zero Balancing Practitioner and Instructor, Santa Cruz, CA

Elson Haas, M.D., Director, Preventive Medical Centers of Marin and Sonoma, San Rafael and Cotati, CA

Jon Kaiser, M.D., private practice, San Francisco, CA

Introduction

The era of Rudyard Kipling—"East is east and west is west, and never the twain shall meet"—is over.

The Western tradition of medicine, built up strongly since the late nineteenth century, has certainly demonstrated that scientific methodologies can deal with illnesses that for centuries had been considered hopeless. Whether we focus on surgery or pharmacology, each of us has personal experiences where people close to us have survived what not long ago would have been certain death at an early age.

In my own family my brother is alive after open heart surgery more than twenty years ago. My wife, stricken with breast cancer more than fifteen years ago, is alive after massive chemotherapy. Children stricken with infectious diseases no longer have to die, as my young cousin did, of streptococcal sore throat.

The successes of conventional medicine range from diseases of the young to the old. Our lives have been affected by it positively in numerous spheres across the life cycle, from birth to death.

However, there is a caveat. The many advances of Western medicine have inadvertently led to new problems. For example, living longer allows more time for the development of chronic and degenerative diseases. "Iatrogenic" problems—illnesses caused by medicine itself—as well as chronic illnesses have forced us to turn toward other dimensions of care, prevention, and health promotion. We are now borrowing from other areas. We are becoming collaborative.

Modern medicine finds itself in a period of profound change. Concepts from other disciplines are quickly being integrated. Most interesting have been those that have come from other cultures—the East and the southern hemisphere. Many treatments we are now familiar with have come from other traditions. Aspirin and quinine are but two that have been westernized by science. More and more such treatments are being transferred and integrated.

Systemic, multidisciplinary, and holistic concepts are now part and parcel of modern medicine. They have either emerged from or developed parallel with long-standing unconventional practices. All this is taking place within a rapidly changing scene.

The New Collaboration

This book opens the door to look at today's predominant alternative medical traditions. Fortunately, it is not an attempt to replace Western medicine. Indeed, as we look carefully into the behavior of mainstream culture as well as our many diverse populations, we find a pattern of mixed use of conventional and unconventional practices.

Introduction

A group of my students studying the Chinese community found that the population was able to separate the need for Western and non-Western care. They consciously chose one or the other depending upon the condition. Western medicine was the clear leader in infectious disease, some cancers, and heart disease.

However, in the ordinary complaints of life—the aches and pains of joints, bones, and muscles—they turned to Chinese medicine practitioners. They found that chronic conditions and their side effects were more judiciously helped by this tradition.

When my wife was treated with chemotherapy for breast cancer we depended upon the best and most advanced protocols of treatment. For the side effects we used antioxidants (now accepted, but then in the netherworld of strange practices), acupuncture, and *chi kung*. We turned to different healers as needed. Like many others, we found that conventional medicine was important and excellent but that it ignored certain issues due to both lack of time and the awareness that they were important. Thus the alternative practitioners supplemented conventional medicine. As a team they were formidable.

Current developments at the National Institutes of Health, where support is now given to the study and implementation of unconventional practices, are encouraging this newfound cooperation. Similarly, in China the training of the two differing kinds of practitioners (Chinese and Western) in each other's practices has led to a better use of resources. Wherever funding and resources are expensive or in short supply, less expensive indigenous healing practices work for large numbers of people.

What we are learning from other cultures has changed conventional medical practice. The importance of the extended family and networks of friends, which is part of life in the non-Western world, has become part of our new knowledge. In epidemiological studies, it has been shown that people who are connected with and supported by others get sick less often, get well faster, and live longer. Those who continue to have meaningful lives in their community live longer than those who retire and just play.

Old people do better when they live with younger ones. Old people whose lives are facilitated by systems that work smoothly—in housing, eating, medical care, education, and general well-being—do better than those in nursing homes or hospitals.

We are also learning from the other health care traditions that have grown up within our own backyard. Natural noninvasive therapies, manipulative therapies, and mind/body approaches are coming of age and taking on a partnership role in relation to Western medicine, impacting it for the better. They can no longer be considered suspect when the evidence of their contributions is so overwhelmingly clear.

Conventional medicine has learned much about the complexity of human biology. It has learned less about how to cope and adapt to crises. Learning from other traditions and the emergence of more ecological, environmental, and psychosocial understanding are leading to a more holistic approach.

Health is the ability to command events that affect your life. It is competence and learning how to cope with stresses and crises, both as individuals and as groups or communities.

The *Healthy Cities* movement, a community networking effort initiated by the World Health Organization to improve the quality of life in the world's urban centers, is demonstrating worldwide that a balanced health system is the only answer. To achieve that balance requires not just scientific medicine, but the awareness of the impact of the complex world on each of our lives. Today over 1,800 cities are participating in this movement, sharing information about how to bring health awareness into all the activities of urban life.[1]

Each of us is unique. We carry different as well as similar genetic patterns. Our life experiences cause us to develop differently. We are people of multiple cultures and practices. Clearly, a total, noncontrolling, almost anarchic approach to living is emerging. This within a sense of community is essential.

Introduction

The joining together of conventional and alternative traditions may well permit us to have a more balanced quality of life. At the least, it has helped to bring the concept of health back to medicine.

Len Duhl, M.D., Professor
School of Public Health
The University of California, Berkeley

CHAPTER 1

THE CRISIS OF FREEDOM: HOW DO WE CHOOSE?

"Surely every medicine is an innovation; and he that will not apply new remedies must expect new evils; for time is the greatest innovator."

—FRANCIS BACON (1625)

Martin is a forty-five-year-old father, husband, and school-teacher who has been suffering from an uncomfortable and sometimes painful prostate condition. He has heard about the growing epidemic of prostate cancer with news reports of senators, a supreme court justice, a former president, and other celebrities. He has also heard that prostate cancer is striking at progressively younger ages, that one in eleven men will be affected, and that all men over forty should be checked regularly. He is worried that his condition might be precancerous or worse.

His urologist (a specialist in disorders of the urinary and genital systems) recommended a prostate specific antigen (PSA) test to rule out cancer. The PSA test, an important recent advance of conventional (allopathic) medicine, is a $60 blood test that allows the early detection of cancer or precancerous conditions.

Martin was relieved to hear his test results were negative. After a thorough examination, the urologist gave him the diagnosis of noninfectious congestive prostatitis, telling him that his condition is not caused by infection and that the cause is unknown. He offered Martin a prescription for an anti-inflammatory drug, which he said happens to be mixed with an antibiotic. When Martin inquired about why he would be taking an antibiotic, his doctor said, "That's just the way the drug comes. It won't hurt you."

The urologist also gave him a list of foods and beverages called "GU irritants" (chocolate, coffee, citrus fruits, pineapples, tomatoes, strawberries, condiments, nuts, spices, and alcohol). Further, he suggested Martin may benefit from more sexual activity and perhaps return visits for prostate massage.

On the way home, Martin began to wonder what help might be available from some other forms of medicine. He appreciated the expertise of his urologist, yet he wondered if there was in fact a cause that could be identified. The thought of being dependent on medication and office visits for prostate massage was disquieting, as was the idea of having to avoid some of his favorite foods.

And, indeed, he does have choices. He could seek the counsel of a naturopathic physician. In naturopathy, inflammatory and congestive conditions are believed to be related to the body's inability to eliminate a burden of toxins that have accumulated in its tissues from the environment or improper diet. The naturopath might recommend a detoxification program, evaluate his diet, and explain the need for essential fatty acids, amino acids, certain vitamins, and zinc for the prostate. There may also be recommendations of herbal remedies, like saw palmetto, ginseng, or flower pollen extracts, and hydrotherapy in the form of a sitz bath alternating hot and cold water.

Martin could also go to a practitioner of Chinese medicine, who might recommend a series of acupuncture treatments to stimulate and harmonize the flow of *chi*, or life force energy, throughout the body. He may be told that his prostate condition represents a pooling or a stagnation of energy in the prostate region, and that this is symptomatic of a larger systemic problem in the flow of energy through his body. In addition to the acupuncture, some Chinese herbs might be recommended to reduce

2

the congestion. He might be advised to *reduce* sexual activity, since it may further irritate his prostate and deplete his *chi*. Finally, he may receive instruction in certain *chi kung* practices, a form of meditation and breathing exercises that he can do on his own to further work with the flow of his energy.

Martin could also go to a classical homeopath who, after a single exhaustive, detailed interview, might prescribe a remedy in pill form that would provoke his body's healing responses to a higher level. Ideally this would be a onetime, one-dose treatment. It would work by stimulating his body's innate healing resources to eliminate the prostate congestion. He might be told to expect a temporary increase of symptoms as his body adjusts to the remedy before the symptoms disappear. This treatment may not bring immediate relief, but it may bring a more enduring cure in the long run.

He could go to a practitioner of Ayurveda and have his *dosha*, or mind/body type—*pitta, kapha,* or *vata*—diagnosed. The Ayurvedic practitioner might, based on further tongue and pulse diagnosis, recommend a more appropriate diet for him based specifically on his *dosha*, along with certain Ayurvedic herbs and beverages. He may be instructed to massage certain points on his feet and ankles with castor oil, massage his perineum, practice certain yoga postures each day, meditate, and avoid sex since that would cause further irritation and contribute to more congestion of energy in his prostate.

Martin might suspect the prostatitis is stress related and go to a practitioner of behavioral or mind/body medicine for stress reduction or psychotherapy. He might undergo training in the relaxation response and mental imagery to encourage his body's healing responses. Hypnotherapy might also be suggested to help him discover what his body—and his prostate—might be saying to him about his lifestyle. The practitioner may also recommend that he get more physical exercise to release tension and build fitness, and shorten the periods each day in which he is sitting.

He could visit a chiropractor who might use a series of spinal adjustments and manipulations to work with the nerve supply from the spine to the prostate region. The chiropractor may explain that Martin's sedentary lifestyle may contribute to problems in the spine and lower back area, in turn affecting the nerve supply to the prostate region. If the nerve supply is in any way being interfered with by spinal disorders, then the body's natural healing processes will be unable to handle the prostate condition, resulting in chronic and perhaps degenerative problems. Several adjustments and certain stretching exercises for the spine may be recommended.

Martin could consult with a practitioner of osteopathic medicine who might perform similar treatments to those of the chiropractor. In addition, since an osteopath is licensed to prescribe medication, Martin may be advised to take a prescription medication, have other treatments similar to those offered by an allopathic physician, or even take a naturopathic remedy.

Finally, he could choose a form of bodywork or massage. He may consider a series of Rolfing sessions. Rolfing is a form of deep tissue manipulation that releases adhesions of the fascia, the tissue that surrounds and encapsulates the muscles and organs of the body. By releasing stuck places in the fascia, the flow of energy, blood circulation, and nerve impulses throughout the body are improved. Martin might also consider a practitioner of acupressure massage, a form of oriental massage that works to stimulate and harmonize the flow of *chi* through the body by stimulating and manipulating certain points on the acupuncture meridians but without needles.

Each of the above traditions has its own unique perspective on Martin's condition. Each has its strengths and limitations, and as we shall see throughout this book, each is increasingly coming under scientific scrutiny to establish its efficacy. Still, he alone must choose.

HOW DO WE CHOOSE?

The choices we have are among forms of medicine that sometimes appear to compete with and even contradict one another. One tradition's medicine may literally be another's poison. Our choice of medical care also makes a statement about what we believe our relationship is to our health and perhaps even to life in a broader sense.

There are several factors that can influence our decision. To many of us, dealing with any kind of medicine is intimidating. Having choices to make is met with a feeling of trepidation because we feel so unprepared. We have been taught that medical matters are the province of authorities outside ourself. We may have the feeling that "the fewer choices I have to make, the better."

Often the easiest path is simply to follow our family history, using the tradition with which we grew up. For most westerners, of course, this would mean allopathic medicine, and this is likely to be a comfortable decision because the allopathic tradition has historically encouraged this placement of authority, recommendations, and decisions about what is best for us in the hands of the practitioner.

Others may take a more introspective approach and base their choice on philosophical or even religious considerations. Two of the traditions we will be examining, Chinese medicine and Ayurveda, have strong associations with religious or spiritual belief systems. Indeed, these systems view themselves as broader than just forms of medicine, but rather as an entire way of life. The influences of Eastern thought, with the notion of health as a matter of living in harmony and balance in all areas of life—spiritually, emotionally, and physically—are integral to these traditions.

Someone else may base their choice not on the tradition itself, but rather on the personal relationship with a practitioner. You may ask your friends for a recommendation of a practitioner with whom you would feel comfortable. You may believe that what is most important is not the form of medicine, but the fact that you are working with someone whom you feel you can trust, who takes time to listen, offers warmth, who is empathic, and, perhaps most of all, who cares. Many would argue that the interpersonal relationship between practitioner and patient is the most potent form of medicine of all and is more important than any other treatment.

Some of us are limited in our choice by purely economic considerations. Those who must depend upon insurance coverage or government programs may find a very narrow range of freedom of choice, usually limited to the allopathic tradition because it is so deeply institutionalized in our society. Ironically, nonallopathic forms of medicine tend to be less costly and more prevention oriented than allopathy. Some insurance companies and government agencies are showing a new openness to these alternatives given the long-range economics and limited success of allopathy with many conditions.

Proximity is another factor for some. The large population centers have the greatest availability of the full range of medical traditions. Historically this has meant that people outside these areas are usually limited to allopathy, although this is changing. As nonallopathic traditions gain greater acceptance their availability is expanding beyond the large urban centers.

Finally, some consider the question of scientific support. The government and its regulatory agencies have asserted for decades that scientific evidence should be the basis of evaluation for all forms of medicine. While such evidence has been slow in coming, particularly for the nonallopathic traditions, consumers are showing themselves to be increasingly sophisticated in their demands for objective information. Popular health and news magazines now place high value on news of scientific evidence for alternative forms of medicine.

ART OR SCIENCE? THE QUEST FOR A "SCIENTIFIC MEDICINE"

In 1992 the mainstreaming of alternative medicine took a quantum leap when Congress mandated the creation of the Office of Alternative Medicine at the National Institutes of Health. This office is charged with evaluating and disseminating information about the effectiveness, strengths, and limitations of nonallopathic forms of medicine.

This task is complicated by the fact that the practice of medicine is an art rather than a science. The encounter between practitioner and patient is, after all, a relationship between two human beings, each with his or her unique sensitivities, expectancies, perceptions, and intuitive awareness. These subjective variables assure that each meeting is itself unique. The practice of medicine can, however, be a *science-based* art. That is, it can be based on principles that have been, at least to some degree, scientifically studied.

Various medical traditions differ in how much their principles have been validated by Western scientific methods. Allopathy aspires to the highest degree of science-based practice. However, its practice is not as scientifically based as many would hope. According to professor David Eddy of Duke University Medical School, 80 percent of allopathy is not governed by scientific data. When researchers studied the consistency of practice across the country, they found major variations in the rates of certain procedures that could not be explained on the basis of population differences. The conclusion was that doctors in different regions of the country practice very differently for no reason except that they had different opinions or habits.

Ayurveda and Chinese medicine evolved long before the Western philosophy of science and principles of empiricism coalesced into what today we call the scientific method. Hence, scientific scrutiny under Western standards has not been a major part of their traditions.

Some of their proponents have expressed the belief that Western science can never adequately study them because of their complexity and subtlety. Instead they often cite these traditions' thousands of years of experience as the evidence of their efficacy. Their perspective is that the principles have been refined and tested continuously down through the ages and, as a result, are tried and true.

The critics of course would respond that only systematic study can bring a practice from the realm of folk medicine to scientific medicine, and that just because a practice is thousands of years old does not make it valid. Certainly, myths or even mistakes can be codified and institutionalized. How do we know whether

7

the benefits, when they occur, are not simply the result of the power of expectation—precisely *because* the tradition is so old?

The practitioners, convinced by personal experience, may reply that the tradition stands on its own and does not need anyone's approval. They may even feel affronted at the suggestion that such a well-established tradition should be questioned now.

The reality is that we live in a society that values sound scientific findings. Doubt and questioning are the basis of the scientific method. The gold standard in scientific practice is of course the arduous double-blind, placebo-controlled clinical trial. However, this is a difficult method to employ, especially for traditions that aim to treat the whole person rather than a specific disease or symptom.

There need to be, and indeed there are, a variety of other ways to objectively establish the credibility of a tradition. In fact, a recent statement by the NIH reflected this view, saying, "Not all alternative medical practices are amenable to traditional scientific evaluation, and some may require development of new methods to evaluate their efficacy and safety."[1]

It is possible to measure the effects of many substances, techniques, and procedures used in nonallopathic traditions. It is certainly possible to measure changes in many symptoms and in the chemistry of bodily fluids that reveal general, if not specific, aspects of health status. Treatment outcomes of course are really the most important criteria for evaluation, and there is nothing that would preclude a well-planned study from comparing treatment outcomes among medical alternatives. This kind of study is in the offing now that NIH is showing fresh interest in evaluating unconventional forms of medicine.

While some of the more conservative forces in nonmainstream traditions may still scoff at the request for scientific evaluation, there is now a growing consensus that it is valuable and worth pursuing. It makes good publicity, it is good for business, and it is possible to do. Each form of medicine discussed in this book has undergone at least some of this kind of scrutiny. Consider the following examples of research findings, all of which were derived using conventional scientific methods:

- A controlled study of patients with allergic asthma found significantly reduced symptoms and better respiratory functioning in those receiving a homeopathic remedy.[2]
- Certain herbs used in Ayurveda have been found to be highly effective free radical scavengers and to reduce rates of tumor growth in rat and human cell systems.[3]
- Acupuncture has been found to increase immune cell counts and trigger a release of substances that promote healing and reduce pain.[4]
- Two naturopathic remedies, zinc supplementation and the herb saw palmetto, have been found to reduce prostate disorders.[5,6] Increasingly, natural substances such as taxol, a product of the Pacific yew tree, are being studied and used in cancer treatment.
- In mind/body medicine, training in the relaxation response has been found to significantly improve immune functioning[7] and group therapy has been found to extend survival time in metastatic breast cancer.[8]

MAKING SENSE OF RESEARCH

How do we evaluate such findings? One of the keys to understanding scientific results is to know the meaning of the term "significance." When studies report significant effects, this usually means that a *statistically* significant change was found (for example, increased natural killer cell activity). This tells us that some real effect was indeed happening and the results are not just a fluke. But this is not the same as saying the effects were *clinically* significant. That is, the effects may or may not be of a magnitude that would actually affect the course of a person's illness.

For example, finding that an herbal substance increases natural killer cell activity in the laboratory is cause for hope. It tells us that there are pathways of influence and potentials to be explored, but it does *not* tell us its real impact on an illness or to what degree this substance would prolong a person's life. On the other hand, the finding in the Stanford study that group therapy nearly doubled the survival time of metastatic breast cancer patients is obviously a clinically significant finding.

Hence, as the more newly established forms of medicine increase the scientific testing of their principles, the real gold medals will go to the studies that can demonstrate clinical significance. Since they involve human subjects, these kinds of studies have much greater ethical and logistical demands and so are more difficult and costly to carry out, but they go the farthest in establishing the credibility of the tradition.

ON THE HORIZON: OUTCOME RESEARCH

In comparing alternative forms of medicine, the most meaningful kind of studies will be those in which the outcomes of several traditions are compared in treating groups of patients with the same illness. A major challenge to this will be getting the traditions to agree on the pool of patients to be compared since the means of diagnosis, and even diagnostic categories, vary from one tradition to the next. It may be necessary for such a sample of patients to be selected using the criteria of one tradition, such as allopathy, for a specific illness, such as influenza.

This kind of study will go a long way toward clarifying the relative effectiveness of different traditions with particular illnesses. Such outcome research is in fact part of the mission of the new Office of Alternative Medicine at NIH.

THE BENEFITS OF DIVERSITY

A great benefit of the new diversity in the medical marketplace is that researchers from all traditions are beginning to conduct studies closely examining the principles and treatments and to publish their findings in scientific journals. Data has persuasive power. The common language and methods of scientific investigation clarify the unique contributions of the various traditions.

This in turn is bringing them wider understanding and acceptance. Ultimately, it will reveal the unique strengths of different forms of medicine and how they can be integrated. Such integration offers perhaps our greatest hope for mastering the difficult challenges confronting us now and in the future.

AN ITINERARY

The remainder of this book is devoted to the exploration of the predominant alternative health care traditions available today. By "tradition" I mean a relatively coherent, organized body of principles and practices for addressing a wide range of health concerns. Each tradition has its own heritage—its own "worldview" for understanding you, your health, and your symptoms.

The crisis of freedom that we face is the challenge of choosing wisely in an environment where we have many options but little help in understanding them. To that end, I have developed a set of questions that will guide this inquiry. The questions will help clarify the essential differences among traditions and can be used as guidelines for making an informed choice. Certain questions will be more important to you than others. Through exploring these issues, you will get an intuitive sense of what feels right for you.

For each tradition we will consider:

1. Key principles: What underlying theories, principles, or beliefs guide this tradition's understanding of health and illness?
2. Variations within the tradition: Are there different forms of practice or specialties within this tradition? How are they identified?

11

3. Procedures and techniques: What kinds of procedures and techniques am I most likely to encounter?

4. Scientific support: What scientific evidence is there to support this tradition's methods, principles, and effectiveness?

5. Strengths and limitations: With what kinds of illnesses is this tradition most and least effective?

6. The practitioner-patient relationship: What kind of personal attention and support can I expect from a practitioner?

7. Evaluating personal results: How will my progress and the effectiveness of my treatment be evaluated? Are there objective measures or tests?

8. Relationship to other forms of medicine: Does this tradition exclude other forms of medicine? Will it interfere or can I combine it with another tradition?

9. Costs: How expensive are consultations, procedures, and medicines? What about insurance coverage?

10. Choosing a practitioner: What credentials should I look for in choosing a practitioner of this tradition?

Within each chapter numerous case examples of the use of the tradition with a variety of conditions will be presented.

CHAPTER 2

CHINESE MEDICINE: THE COSMIC SYMPHONY

"Heaven, Earth, and I are living together, and all things
and I form an inseparable unity."
                                        —CHUANG TZU

Chinese medicine has treated many hundreds of millions of
people over the last three thousand years. It entered the United
States in the 1700s with physicians who were trained in France
and in the 1800s with practitioners from the Orient. It was
embraced to some degree by American mainstream medicine
early in this century, as evidenced by references to the successful
treatment of sciatica and lumbago by acupuncture in H. Gray's
Anatomy, Descriptive and Surgical (1901 edition) and W.
Osler's *The Principles and Practice of Medicine* (1892–1947
editions).

An estimated nine to twelve million patient visits per year are
made to practitioners of Chinese medicine in the United States,
most seeking acupuncture for treatment of pain symptoms after
unsatisfactory results with Western medicine.[1] There are between nine and ten thousand practitioners of acupuncture,[2] in-

13

cluding about three thousand physicians who have varying amounts of training in continuing education programs through American medical schools.[3]

Thirty-five schools of Chinese medicine in the United States now train nonphysician practitioners in programs lasting three to four years. In 1973 Nevada became the first state to license nonphysician practitioners of acupuncture. Twenty-three states restrict the practice of acupuncture to physicians only, while the remainder have varying degrees of regulation for nonphysicians.

To the westerner, perhaps Chinese medicine's most striking quality is its differentness from our conventional ways of thinking. This applies to its views of what health is, what causes health and illness, how healing occurs, and the language used to describe all this. In fact, it may seem that to understand Chinese medicine one needs to learn a different language. And, indeed, as we shall see, even within Chinese medicine there are different vocabularies.

Chinese medicine is actually a blanket term for several different but related traditions of healing. They trace their roots to the time of the Han Dynasty about two thousand years ago and beyond. This was the golden age of philosophy, culture, and medicine in China. An important product of the era was an effort by seven scholars of medicine to unify the society's medical practices. They compiled *The Nei Jing*, also known as *The Yellow Emperor's Classic of Internal Medicine*. This book was an attempt to describe the many diverse and even contradictory views of healing that had existed in China up to that time.

KEY PRINCIPLES

Chinese medicine is a nature-based paradigm of medicine. Nature and the laws that govern the natural or outer world are used to help us understand the inner world, the world of the body. The person is seen as a microcosm of a holographic universe. Thus Chinese medicine offers a cosmological perspective, one in which the person is viewed as an ecosystem embedded in and related to the larger ecosystem around us and governed by the same basic laws.

Yin and Yang

At the foundation of Chinese medical theory is the concept of yin-yang. Just as there are cycles of day and night, the ebb and flow of ocean tides, and the changing of the seasons, human health is also a function of ever-changing patterns of energy constantly seeking harmony and balance. The principle of yin-yang captures this dynamic interplay.

Yin is sometimes described as the feminine principle and yang the masculine. All of life is somehow an expression of the interplay between yin and yang. Every physiological process and symptom can be analyzed in the light of yin-yang theory. Since the ultimate goal of Chinese medicine is to balance and strengthen (tonify), every form of treatment has, in a broad sense, one of the following aims:

To tonify yang
To tonify yin
To eliminate excess yang
To eliminate excess yin[4]

The Vivifying Force: *Chi* (*Qi*)

Yin and yang are complementary aspects of another concept at the heart of Chinese medicine, *chi* (sometimes also spelled *qi*). We have no equivalent word in English. Roughly translated as "life force energy" or "life activity," *chi* is more than just energy as we think of it in Western terms—as, for example, horsepower

15

or wattage. Rather, *chi* has the qualities of life itself. As described by San Francisco practitioner Efrem Korngold, L.Ac., *chi* is what makes life possible, suggesting a biodynamic quality of action or movement. *Chi* is the intangible force that animates us and makes us alive. All that is alive has *chi* and what is not alive has no *chi*.[5]

The diverse traditions or schools within Chinese medicine have different languages for describing the action and qualities of *chi*, but the common principle is that *chi* flows through the body and enlivens it. Health is a function of a balanced, harmonious flow of *chi* and illness results when there is a blockage or imbalance in the flow of *chi*.

The human being has pathways called meridians through which the *chi* flows. The body has been mapped with these meridians, which pass through all its organs. Specific meridians correspond with specific organs or organ systems (organ networks). Health is an ongoing process of maintaining balance among all the organs and systems of the body.

The Meaning of Symptoms

Symptoms are seen as signals of trouble somewhere in the flow of *chi*. To only remove a symptom would be like removing a flashing generator light from your car's dashboard because you are annoyed by it when what it is doing is signaling to you the presence of a deeper problem.

Symptoms are considered as part of a larger picture or pattern affecting the whole person. The practitioner seeks to connect seemingly unrelated symptoms and come up with a unifying explanation in terms of what is going on with the person's *chi* on a global basis. This of course is opposite to the allopathic approach (conventional Western medicine) with its use of specialists for different symptoms and different parts of the body.

In the words of San Francisco acupuncturist Harriet Beinfield,

Barbara

Barbara is a thirty-six-year-old woman who had been diagnosed five years previously with endometrial cancer. During this period she had been treated with chemotherapy (Adriamycin), which produced cardio-myopathy (heart damage). As a result, she developed mild congestive heart failure. She had shortness of breath and could not lie down flat on her bed. She also had a creatinine level of 4.9, which indicated that her kidneys were not functioning well.

She was scheduled for more chemo but both these conditions had made her ability to withstand the stresses of another round tenuous. She sought help from Chinese medicine to prepare herself because her oncologist felt that she was not a good candidate for it at this time.

Barbara began having acupuncture once a week and taking Chinese herbal extracts three times daily with hot water. The herbs were for the purpose of strengthening her heart and kidneys and improving the relationship between them. After three weeks her creatinine level had gone down to 2.3, which was the lowest it had been in two years, indicating that her kidney function had improved markedly. She also came out of congestive heart failure and could lie down flat on the table. After a month she was strong enough to qualify for chemotherapy.

According to acupuncturist Harriet Beinfield, "What Chinese medicine can do is not necessarily attack the disease, which in this case is cancer, but improve the function of the organs and the general health of the body, which includes the immune system. The disease and the chemotherapy had degraded her general health and the functioning of her organs. We were able to boost their function by administering treatments that particularly nourished the systems that were degraded."

L.Ac.: "When people come to Chinese medicine they find one person who understands how their back problem is connected to their abdominal distension, which is connected to the dryness in their eyes, which is connected to their sometimes aggressive and sometimes passive feelings. All the symptoms the person may experience become integrated, which enables them to feel like one whole person who is seeking guidance from another for help with all the parts of themselves."[6]

Treatment of Illness

When illness arises, the practitioner thinks in terms of different qualities of the person's *chi* and what the *chi* is doing as it moves through the person—for example, it may be stagnating or blocked in a certain place, or it may be deficient or excessive. To correct these dysfunctions, the main treatments work directly with the flow of *chi*. The vocabulary of such work often includes such verbs as *tonify, consolidate, replenish, comfort, disperse, purge, strengthen,* and *harmonize.* In Western terms, the goals of treatment are very much in alignment with our concept of strengthening "host resistance," the body's defenses and overall ability to resist disease.

Perspective on Modern Health Problems

Most modern diseases are considered *chi*-deficiency diseases, caused by our not maintaining or supporting a harmonious internal ecology. Chronic stress and tension deplete our inner resources and impair the flow of *chi* through our organ networks. Our poor diet denies the nourishment needed to keep the organ systems healthy so they can do their part in helping maintain balance. Our sedentary lifestyle further promotes the stagnation of our vital energy, with poor circulation and the accumulation of toxins in our tissues.

When our *chi* is depleted or blocked we become more vulnerable to infection by viruses, bacteria, or other organisms. And we are more vulnerable to the degenerative processes that our society has come to associate with normal aging.

Because of our interconnectedness with the environment around us, the worldwide ecological crises occurring at this time are especially problematic for our health. As acupuncturist David Walker, L.Ac., of Santa Rosa, California, puts it, the erosion or mismanagement of the terrain around us makes it more difficult for our inner terrain to maintain its vitality. "How can you be well living in a sea of toxicity?"[7]

VARIETIES OF CHINESE MEDICINE

Chinese medicine is rich with many varieties and traditions. There is no systematic way to categorize them because they differ in so many dimensions. Some variations are defined by their specific methods. Others are defined geographically, ethnically, or politically. Since its influence spread throughout Asia long before it ever came to the West, it permeated many different cultures. Today varieties of it are part of Japanese, Korean, and several Southeast Asian cultures.

The term "oriental medicine" is commonly used to encompass the various traditions that trace their historic roots to Chinese medicine. However, in this book I will stick with the term "Chinese" in order to avoid confusion with Ayurveda, a distinct tradition from India which many people also think of as part of the Orient. Following are descriptions of the major forms most people are likely to encounter in the West today.

Anne

Anne is a thirty-seven-year-old woman who had been diagnosed a year earlier with multiple sclerosis. She sought help with weariness, fatigue, and sometimes clumsiness and disequilibrium. She began a regimen of acupuncture once a week along with a formula of herbal extracts.

Within a month she felt her energy level dramatically increase to where she did not feel tired in the afternoon, could stay up later at night, and could increase the activities that she had cut back on over the previous year.

According to Harriet Beinfield, the treatment served to replenish the Kidney system and *jing*, or "essence."

Traditional Chinese Medicine (TCM)

In the 1940s and 50s the government of communist China undertook an effort to coalesce the myriad forms of Chinese medicine into a unified system called traditional Chinese medicine (TCM). Their intent was a practical one: to integrate a large workforce of traditional practitioners into Western-style hospital medicine as a way of providing care for a large population with inexpensive and familiar methods. Contrary to what its name implies, TCM is actually a modern system and was not an idealistic effort to preserve one particular tradition.

Practitioners of TCM outnumber those of other forms of Chinese medicine in the United States. Most American schools teach this approach. The majority of practitioners are Caucasians who studied here, though many have undergone short internships in China.

The theoretical basis of TCM is the Eight Principles. These are actually four pairs of complementary opposites that describe the *patterns* of disharmony within the person. Briefly the principles are *interior/exterior*, referring to the location of the disharmony in the body (internal organs versus skin or bones); *hot/cold*, referring to qualities of the disease pattern, such as fever or thirst versus chilliness or desire to drink warm liquids; *full/empty*, referring to whether the condition is acute or chronic and whether the body's responses are strong or weak; and the balance of *yin/yang*, which adds further to the description of the other six principles.

TCM places a heavy emphasis on herbal medicine, which is supplemented by acupuncture. For many people this is practical in that they can treat themselves on a daily basis with their herbal remedies and not have to rely on office visits for acupuncture. However, using both methods together is considered the ideal.

Five Element Acupuncture

Also known as classical acupuncture, Five Element acupuncture is the longest established form of Chinese medicine in the United States. Its philosophy is that acupuncture (without herbs) is a complete medical system in itself. As David Walker explains, "Acupuncture itself is a complicated enough art to master, and herbal medicine is another whole study. To do justice to both in the same lifetime would be very difficult."

Many Western practitioners are trained according to the curriculum developed by J. R. Worsley, who founded the College of Traditional Acupuncture in Leamington Spa, England. The theory of the Five Elements—fire, earth, metal, water, and wood—pervades the teaching, philosophy, and methods of traditional acupuncture. The Five Elements are conceived of not just as basic constituents of matter, but as dynamic qualities of nature. They have been called "further descriptions of the *chi* energy as it goes through cyclic transformations. Everything in life is concordant with these elements. . . ."[8]

As *chi* circulates through us it is influenced by the elements as they build upon each other and support each other in a certain orderly *sequence*: wood creates fire, fire creates earth, earth creates metal, metal creates water, and water creates wood. Hence, according to Dianne Connelly, "Health is the harmonious balanced cyclic interaction of these elements. Health is maintained only when the energy flowing through each of the elements is clear and lifegiving."[9]

Each of the body's five organ networks corresponds with a particular element: Heart/Small Intestine with fire, Spleen/Stomach with earth, Lungs/Large Intestine with metal, Kidneys/Bladder with water, and Liver/Gallbladder with wood. The practitioner's efforts to harmonize the Five Elements promote greater harmony in the functioning of all the organ networks.

Medical Acupuncture

It is somewhat awkward to include a discussion of medical acupuncture in a chapter on Chinese medicine since it involves the importation of acupuncture techniques into the practice of Western medicine, an altogether different tradition. Because of its origins, however, we will discuss it here.

Medical acupuncture is the practice of acupuncture performed by a Western-trained allopathic physician (M.D.) or osteopathic physician (D.O.). At this writing, twenty-three states allow only this kind of acupuncture.

Medical acupuncture developed in Europe as a result of the introduction of Chinese medical texts and practices by traders and missionaries in the seventeenth and eighteenth centuries. It has evolved alongside allopathic medicine in Europe where it is taught in many medical schools and used in most fields of medicine. In the United States, training programs for physicians were first offered in the late 1970s, and

22

by the mid-1980s medical acupuncture emerged as a medical discipline.

Most practitioners are already established in a conventional medical specialty and use acupuncture in that context. It serves as an adjunct technique as opposed to being considered a complete medical system in itself.

According to Joseph Helms, M.D., founding president of the American Academy of Medical Acupuncture and coordinator of physician education in acupuncture, Office of Continuing Education, UCLA School of Medicine, the practitioners tend to use a hybrid approach to acupuncture, taking the strengths of as many approaches to acupuncture as possible and integrating them into the context of Western medicine. Hence, they may draw upon the Eight Principles used in TCM, the Five Elements approach of classical acupuncture, and other systems.

Medical acupuncture conceives of the therapeutic mechanisms of acupuncture in the neurophysiologic and bioelectric terms familiar to Western science, as well as the energetic models derived from the classical texts.

The American Medical Association does not yet recognize acupuncture as a specialty or a special technique of medicine.

Ethnic Chinese Traditional Medicine

This is a more loosely defined, generic form of Chinese medicine and is usually practiced by the ethnic Chinese in large urban centers in the United States. There is no organized body of theory. Both acupuncture and herbs may be used, and some practitioners use electrical stimulation of the needles.

Some practitioners prepare raw herb formulas and send them home in jars with the client. Others instruct clients in doing so at home. The limited English of some practitioners may create some uneasiness on the part of the consumer as to how much their problems are being understood. Still, many westerners are convinced they are receiving effective treatment.

Japanese Acupuncture

While practitioners of this variety are definitely a minority, Japanese acupuncture is growing in popularity among American acupuncturists. Japanese needles are considerably thinner than others, and as a result are now used by many practitioners of other forms of Chinese medicine because they are thought to be less traumatic for the patient.

Japanese acupuncture theory does not incorporate herbal medicine. The needling techniques are reputed to be more gentle and sensitive than other approaches. According to Daniel Kenner, L.Ac., of Santa Rosa, California, and San Francisco's Meiji College of Oriental Medicine, Japanese-style training places greater emphasis on the practitioner developing "an advanced level of tactile sensitivity in locating points with the fingertips. This allows them to actually feel the *chi* flow and feel blockages of energy that are impalpable to the unpracticed hand." The ideal is to then use the mildest intervention possible while achieving the desired effect.

Auricular Acupuncture

Auricular acupuncture is a technique of treating points exclusively on the ear. The points are chosen by different means—palpation for tenderness, electrode resistance, and using the patient's pulse to locate significant points.

Many of its practitioners consider this approach to be a complete medical system for treating functional and allergic disorders, and often use it exclusive of any other type of practice. It is also used for pain control and to assist in withdrawal from drug and alcohol addiction.

Work with drug withdrawal began in Hong Kong in the 1970s. In recent years a movement has developed in the West to expand this application because of evidence of its effectiveness.

Madeline

Madeline is a seven-year-old girl who had chronic asthma, a chronic cough, and eczema all over her legs. She had just begun using bronchodilators, which her mother said turned her into a "little witch"—she would become very irritable and agitated in response to the medication. She'd had no treatment for the eczema.

Her mother brought her to Chinese medicine to seek help with the behavior and mood problems. Rather than using needles, the practitioner rubbed certain acupuncture points and led her through a visualization. She was seen only once and was also given an herbal formula to take twice daily. Within a few weeks her symptoms began to diminish, and by a nine-month follow-up visit her asthma, cough, and eczema had all cleared up.

According to Harriet Beinfield, "The skin is considered to be the third lung, and in that sense the eczema was connected with the asthma. The herbs that affect the lung also affect the skin. The Lung (organ system) likes to be moist, and when it becomes dry it becomes irritated.

"Irritation can sometimes translate into inflammation, which becomes an 'itis'—like bronchitis. The herbs that were used tend to moisturize and nourish the Lung, as well as help to move the *chi* and open the chest."

Abbreviated training programs in auricular acupuncture are growing for detox technicians, nurses, and physical therapists. Some conventionally trained practitioners question the wisdom of allowing people to practice with this briefer training.

The French neurophysiologist Paul Nogier, M.D., developed

a method called auricular medicine or auriculotherapy, based on neuroendocrine theory rather than Chinese medicine. Like medical acupuncture, it integrates a technique drawn from Chinese medicine into a Western context.

Eclectic

Probably the greatest number of Western practitioners of Chinese medicine would describe themselves as eclectic, at least to some degree, though their original training was in one of the above varieties. Given the richness and unique perspectives of the different models, many borrow from several sources to create their own synthesis that works best for them in their own style of practice. The rationale is expressed well by Helms, who thinks of the various models as being layered on top of one another: "Each case makes sense in a slightly different way—each case makes best sense in one model or another."[10]

PROCEDURES AND TECHNIQUES

Diagnosis

Diagnosis is based upon identifying *patterns* of signs and symptoms. These patterns reflect the condition of the internal organ networks as well as the *chi*. The practitioner will examine skin, complexion, bones, channels, smells, sounds, mental state, preferences, emotions, tongue, pulse, demeanor, and body build. Each of these has its own variety of qualities and nuances that help the practitioner discern patterns that underlie the person's complaints. This approach is summed up in the expression "Inspect the exterior to examine the interior."[11]

Some practitioners arrive at a diagnosis with very little verbal exchange with the person. In situations where the practitioner does not speak English, a rapid assessment may be made and work begun without such communication. Other practitioners may conduct an exhaustive interview, while still others will use written questionnaires to get a thorough picture of the patient's pattern of complaints.

Pulse Diagnosis. One of the more mysterious aspects of Chinese medicine to westerners is pulse diagnosis. In Western medicine the pulse is a very simple thing and is used only to measure heart rate—the number of beats per minute.

In Chinese medicine the pulse provides a whole world of information. The primary use is as an indication of various conditions of *chi* moving through the person's meridians. The condition of all the organ networks is assessed via the pulse.

For example, in TCM the flow of *chi* through each of twelve major meridians can be assessed by the practitioner feeling the pulse at various positions on the wrist (the leg or neck can also be used). There are six basic locations and three depths on each wrist.

Each of these positions can be assessed according to many different qualities that the pulse can have—twenty-eight in TCM, other numbers in other variations of Chinese medicine. While these qualities have esoteric-sounding names such as "floating," "thick," "thin," and so on, they are actually features of each pulse that we could see if we were looking at a sine wave of the pulse on an oscilloscope. The qualities may be such things as how strong each pulsation is, its length, how it trails off, and what kind of activity may be present between pulsations. Just as the Eskimos have a very rich vocabulary for describing many varieties and features of snow, there is a rich vocabulary in Chinese medicine for describing the nature of a person's pulse.

The practitioner can feel the balance and flow of *chi* through the person's meridians and corresponding organs. This is not only of value in diagnosis, but also in measuring progress from one treatment to the next. In addition the practitioner can dis-

Harold

Harold was a twenty-four-year-old man with extreme redness of the skin on his body, particularly his face. He looked like he had a very severe sunburn. Some of his body was scabbed because of itching and he had taken pharmaceuticals for dermatitis, but none of them seemed to help.

He had weekly acupuncture for three months, took a combination of herbs, and was told to modify his diet. He was also told not to eat foods that created internal heat—namely sugar, spices, or fat. He was not to drink alcohol and was to increase his water intake so that he stayed hydrated. He was told to eat a cucumber a day, which is very cooling and moisturizing.

Within two to three months Harold's redness began to recede. His face improved first, followed by the rest of his body, ending with his legs.

In Chinese medicine his problem is understood as too much Heat and not enough Moisture (terms that describe the climate within the body). The herbs that were used release excess Internal Heat and Moisturize and Nourish the Lung system (the skin is the third lung).

According to Harriet Beinfield, "We tried to get rid of something undesirable—in this case, Heat—as well as supply something that does not exist sufficiently—Moisture."

cover weaknesses that would warn of future problems with certain organ systems.

Treatment

Herbs. Herbal medicine probably predates acupuncture and in some settings it is the primary form of treatment. In the context of Chinese medicine, the term "herb" is actually used to describe any natural material of plant, animal, or mineral origin, or any traditional or modern preparation of the natural materials short of preparing an isolated chemical.[12]

The traditional use of herbs is not based on their chemistry as we would understand it. They are selected in order to introduce certain influences or qualities into the body, and to balance or harmonize the dynamics that are currently present and may be involved in disease. Some herbs act like highly concentrated medicinal foods that nourish the organ networks. Thus there is an intimate interaction between the energy qualities of the herbs and of the person, and the herbs serve to influence healing and reharmonizing the organ networks.

Chinese herbs are available in three forms. The most traditional are the raw materials themselves, which are given to the patient who takes them home and boils them up into a beverage. This may take the form of a tea consumed on a daily basis one or more times, much the way a westerner would take allopathic medicines according to a certain schedule.

The second form, a modern development, is where the herbal substances are compressed into tablet form and taken as pills. Obviously much more convenient, this eliminates the time involved in boiling the raw herbs. It also eliminates the smell that can permeate the house as a result of boiling herbs, which can be strong and objectionable to some. The tablets can be difficult to swallow, especially if there is a large number of them, and some people question how well the body breaks down and absorbs substances presented in this form. Practitioners generally reply that the tablets are designed for quick breakdown in the stomach.

Finally there are herbal extracts, also convenient. These are provided in an eyedropper bottle in a concentrated form that is added to hot water and consumed as a tea. The extracts have the advantages of being easier to consume and perhaps easier for the body to assimilate than tablets. Since they are in a liquid form, the extracts also allow greater combinations of herbal substances to be easily mixed, so a unique "cocktail" can be easily designed for an individual patient's needs.

Acupuncture. This involves the insertion of thin, sterile, stainless steel needles into points on the surface of the body to a depth just below the surface of the skin in the epidural layer. Most acupuncturists use disposable needles, while a few use reusable needles that are sterilized.

For some people the insertion is barely noticeable, and for others there is a small pinch, sometimes followed by a sensation of numbness, tingling, ache, warmth, or heaviness. The point locations are determined by the geography of the meridians and acupuncture points on the body as described by Chinese medical theory. In some cases the needles are manually twirled to give more stimulation. A few practitioners use electrical stimulation of the needles (electroacupuncture) to add even more effect.

The practitioner selects points based on the diagnosis and goals of treatment. Usually several different points are needled at the same time while the patient is in a reclining position on a table. The insertions may be for just a few seconds, or they may last from twenty to forty minutes while the patient lies still and rests. Most people find the sessions very relaxing, and it is not uncommon to feel immediate effects and changes in symptoms.

In some variations of Chinese medicine the practitioner remains present with the patient throughout the treatment, continuously checking the pulse and perhaps changing needle positions in response to the ongoing feedback from it. This approach is most common among practitioners of classical or Five Element acupuncture.

Other approaches involve leaving the patient alone to rest quietly. The practitioner may go to treat another patient or to prepare herbal remedies. Practitioners vary in how much

30

importance they place on their own presence during the treatment. Some patients feel more comfortable or more cared for if the practitioner remains with them, while others are comfortable with the coming and going of the practitioner. This is another instance in which the practitioner's style may be something you may want to inquire about in advance.

In China, acupuncture is routinely used for anesthesia. In the famous Bill Moyers television series *Healing and the Mind*, shown nationally in 1993, millions of Americans witnessed a person having brain surgery while conscious and carrying on a conversation—all with the help of acupuncture anesthesia.

Moxibustion. Moxibustion treatment is the burning of the herb moxa (mugwort) on an acupuncture point. Moxa is applied in the form of a fluffy, woollylike material that is rolled up by the fingers into roughly the size of a small pea, placed in position, and then lit, usually with an incense stick. It burns slowly, introducing heat into the acupuncture point, and is removed by the practitioner when the patient is able to feel it become hot, usually after a few seconds.

The use of moxibustion is older than that of needles and there was a time when moxa was considered superior to all other treatments. There are different kinds of moxa and its effects are determined by such factors as its age, how tightly it is packed, how many applications are used on a given point, and its juxtaposition with needles. Also, it can be placed on a bed of salt, ginger, or a slice of garlic on the skin to introduce additional properties or influences into the point.

Moxibustion brings influences, especially heat, into the point that the needle cannot. It may also be placed on the exposed tip of the needle and burned in order to change the temperature gradient of the needle.

Massage (Acupressure, Shiatsu). Acupressure and shiatsu are sometimes called acupuncture without needles. They are variations of massage technique in which a similar geography of points and meridians is used to guide the application of finger pressure rather than the insertion of needles. The aims are simi-

31

lar in terms of stimulating points and influencing the flow of *chi* through the meridians. During the course of an acupuncture session, some practitioners use these methods, which are discussed more thoroughly in Chapter 9.

Chi Kung. *Chi kung* (also spelled *qi gong*) is the mother of all the martial arts. It is estimated that 1.3 *million* residents of Beijing use the practices of this five-thousand-year-old tradition, with tens of millions more nationwide. In Shanghai there is even a hospital devoted to treating cancer with these methods.[13]

Chi kung is the oriental counterpart to Western mind/body medicine and contains elements of meditation, relaxation training, visualization, movement, postures, and breathing exercises. In the Orient it serves both as a form of exercise for physical fitness and a self-healing tool.

The aim is to strengthen and direct the flow of *chi* through the body to promote health and well-being. The benefits require daily practice to accrue. This may mean a routine that takes from twenty to forty minutes per day. Some practitioners of Chinese medicine teach these techniques to their patients, while others will refer them to classes taught by specialists.

SCIENTIFIC SUPPORT

The evaluation of Chinese medicine by Western scientific criteria raises some interesting challenges. One is that *chi*, which is at the heart of this tradition, cannot be measured. Another is that many of the treatments are person-specific rather than symptom-specific or disease-specific.

In other words, two people with the same symptoms may be treated entirely differently based on their own unique inner ecology. The idea of a standardized treatment, as used in Western-style research, contradicts this principle. What could help reestablish balance and harmony within one person may have the opposite effect in the next.

OAM-Funded Studies

The Office of Alternative Medicine, National Institutes of Health, has funded four studies related to Chinese medicine in its first wave of research grants.

Acupuncture and Depression. John J. Allen of the University of Arizona in Tucson is conducting a controlled study to test the effectiveness of acupuncture for treatment of unipolar depression in women. The study uses a person-specific approach to diagnosis and treatment of the patients according to Chinese medicine principles. That is, the women will receive individually tailored acupuncture treatments using points not specific to depression.

Acupuncture and ADHD. In the second study, Neil Sonenklar of Virginia Commonwealth University in Richmond is studying the use of acupuncture point therapy in treatment of ADHD (attention deficit hyperactivity disorder) in children, and comparing it to the effectiveness of the common drug treatment, methylphenidate.

Chi Kung and Reflex Sympathetic Dystrophy. In a controlled study, Wen-Hsien Wu of the University of Medicine and Dentistry of New Jersey, Newark, is examining the effectiveness of *chi kung (qi gong)* in treating patients with late stage reflex sympathetic dystrophy (RSD), a chronic and ultimately disabling disease caused by malfunction of the autonomic nervous system.

Tai Chi and Balance Disorders. Finally, Timothy Hain of Northwestern University is examining the use of tai chi as an alternative treatment for people with balance disorders. Change in such factors as dizziness, falls, and postural sway will be considered in evaluating the effects of an eight-week program of daily practice of this oriental discipline.

The attitude among many practitioners has been that Chinese medicine stands on its own merit and has no need for the stamp of approval of Western science. The implicit assumption has been that over the thousands of years in which the methods have evolved, practitioners have refined their understanding based on case-by-case observation and have communicated this collective wisdom effectively to their students or successors.

With the rise of the information age, however, a surprising amount of research has taken place both in the West and in the Orient. Many studies, particularly with herbs, have found important effects that occur independently of individual differences between people. Such studies are more difficult with acupuncture, but there are some interesting findings with this method as well.

Chinese Herbs

While the use of Chinese herbs clearly is based on a theory of energy medicine, they do lend themselves to Western-style research since they can be studied much like pharmacological substances. Their potential is very well illustrated by the clinical research that has been conducted with cancer and heart disease.

Cancer. In modern China, cancer is the leading cause of death. Practitioners there advocate a combination of Chinese and Western medicine as the optimal cancer treatment, accompanied by diet, exercise, and lifestyle change. The rationale for the use of Chinese herbs is twofold: to attack the tumor and to support and strengthen the patient's immune responses.

Chinese medicine uses over 120 different herbs with cancer, depending on the type of cancer and its cause according to Chinese medical theory. One class of herbs used for centuries is called *fu-zhen* herbs. Recent studies have shown why they have proven successful with a variety of cancers.

One controlled study examined the survival time of patients

George

George, a forty-one-year-old teacher, had been diagnosed with chronic prostatitis and urethritis that long-term antibiotics had not helped. His symptoms included difficult urination and painful ejaculations. After ten acupuncture treatments accompanied by daily herbal formulas, his symptoms disappeared.

In Chinese medicine, prostatitis and urethritis are outcomes of too much Heat (a quality of climate) in the Lower Burner (the lower abdomen and associated organs). The herbs used are cooling to eliminate the adverse climate of excess Heat in the Lower Burner.

with stage II primary liver cancer undergoing chemotherapy or radiation. Twenty-nine of the forty-six patients receiving *fu-zhen* herbs along with radiation or chemotherapy survived at least one year and ten survived for three years. Of the thirty patients who received *only* radiation or chemotherapy, six survived one year and none survived three years.[14]

Other varieties of herbs have been used as well, with the following findings:

Improved survival rates for patients with nasopharyngeal, lung, throat, and breast cancers who used herbs in combination with radiation or chemotherapy, as opposed to conventional treatment alone.[15,16]

No significant drop in white blood counts and platelet counts after three cycles of chemotherapy in a group of eleven breast cancer patients using an herbal treatment.[17]

In 181 patients with precancerous throat lesions, only 9 percent of those treated with herbs developed cancer within five years, as opposed to 26 percent in the untreated group.[18]

White blood counts of forty patients receiving radiotherapy

recovered significantly with herbs, as opposed to a control group whose counts dropped significantly without them.[19]

A study of forty patients with various cancers found an herbal treatment to significantly increase lymphocyte transformation.[20]

In 272 patients with nasopharyngeal cancer, those treated with Chinese herbs and radiation had a significantly lower five-year relapse rate than those with radiation alone (12 percent vs. 38 percent). Five-year survival rates were also higher (67 percent vs. 48 percent).[21]

In 326 patients with postoperative stomach cancer, a significantly higher percentage of those receiving herbal treatment were able to tolerate chemotherapy than those not receiving it (95 percent vs. 79 percent). Other outcomes included improved weight gain, fewer complaints of low energy, and improved natural killer cell activity.[22]

In 158 patients with late-stage stomach cancer, treatment with herbs was associated with significantly higher three-, five-, and ten-year survival rates than normal. Survivors also showed enhanced immune functioning.[23]

Heart Disease. The findings with heart disease include lower oxygen consumption by the heart muscle (indicating less energy required in pumping), dilating the coronary arteries (which increases the blood supply to the heart), reducing angina, lowering blood cholesterol levels, reducing platelet aggregation and adhesion to arteries, increasing contractile force of the heart, increasing cardiac output, and reducing high blood pressure.[24] A few examples of clinical studies include:

A study of thirty-seven patients with coronary heart disease and fourteen with recent heart attacks found an herbal combination to strengthen heart functioning, increase oxygen supply to the myocardium, and inhibit clotting.[25]

A placebo-controlled study of forty-six angina pectoris patients found a reduction of pain of 85 percent for the herbs (versus 37 percent for those not receiving the herbs) and an ECG improvement rate of 45 percent (versus 3 percent).[26]

In 110 coronary heart disease patients, herbal treatment

showed an 81-percent effective rate for angina pectoris, improved ECG in 65 percent, and improved cardiac function in 57 percent, all significant differences to the control group.[27]

A double-blind study of the effect of another herb on sixty-five coronary heart disease patients found reduced symptoms in 73 percent of cases (42-percent improvement with a placebo) and ECG improvement in 60 percent (25-percent improvement with a placebo).[28] The benefits were attributed to increased volume of coronary blood flow, making more oxygen available throughout the heart.

A study of 136 patients with abnormal blood lipid levels found the herb rosa multiflora to be as effective as two common conventional drugs for reducing blood lipids.[29]

A controlled study with seventy-five coronary heart disease patients compared an herbal formula to dextrose and cedilandid-D. The effects of the two treatments were similar in increasing the muscular contractile force and reduced oxygen consumption in the myocardium.[30]

In sixty coronary heart disease patients an herbal formula was found to have positive effects on angina pectoris, blood lipids, and left cardiac function tests.[31]

In 308 patients an herbal oil was tested for its ability to reduce blood lipids. There was a significant decrease, along with reduction in platelet aggregation rates and blood pressure.[32]

Another study randomly divided 430 acute heart attack patients into two groups. One group received conventional drug treatment combined with a formula of six Chinese herbs. The other group received only conventional treatment. The fatality rate for those receiving the herbs was 6.5 percent versus 14.9 percent for the control group.[33]

Finally, a study of 120 cases of coronary heart disease found an herbal treatment to reduce the occurrence of angina pain in 85 percent of patients and improve ECG indices in 77 percent of patients.[34]

It is worth noting that no adverse reactions or side effects were observed in the above studies, many of which used blood, urine, liver, and kidney tests to look for such effects.

Acupuncture

In contrast to herbal medicine, studies of acupuncture are more difficult because the individual artistry of the practitioner is such an important part of the technique and treatment is normally individualized for each patient. Hence there are very few studies that adhere to Western standards.

Proponents of acupuncture argue that to insist on imposing such standards to justify this form of medicine would be to our detriment. According to Joseph Helms, M.D., "Using scientifically proven mechanisms as the exclusive foundation to define acupuncture applications overlooks the heritage of empirical observations by traditional practitioners. To ignore this heritage is to deprive a contemporary physician of models of health, disorder, and treatment that are presented in classical texts, models that have been vitally useful to practitioners in many cultures during the long history of acupuncture."[35]

In other words, the collective wisdom of centuries of practical experience should not be discarded. Rather, it should be embraced as a valuable contribution to modern medicine.

Acupuncture research in the West has dealt mostly with documenting its mechanisms in pain control.[36,37] According to Helms, the mechanisms by which acupuncture reduces pain are in fact "defined more clearly than most drugs, and certainly most analgesic drugs that are commercially in use today."[38]

Physiology of Acupuncture Effects. There is evidence that acupuncture activates the electric system, the nervous system, the blood system, and the lymph system. In terms of pain control, what Western science understands most clearly is that there is a cascade of neurotransmitters that are released as a result of acupuncture stimulation. These are the endorphins, enkaphalins, monoamines, and neurotransmitters that help inhibit pain transmission and reception through the central nervous system. Other mechanisms by which acupuncture can benefit medical conditions remain less clearly understood.

Helms is careful to point out that while the basic science is

Julia

Julia is a fifty-six-year-old woman who was on post-menopausal hormone replacement therapy because of extreme mood swings and hot flashes. Without the therapy she would become quite irritable and fly into rages that she felt were unfair to her children and husband.

Julia sought help from Chinese medicine because of the side effects of the therapy. One was bruising and swelling—for example, if she bumped her elbow her whole arm would swell up. Another was water retention; she increased half a dress size and the rings on her fingers were uncomfortably tight. She wanted to see if she could find an alternative to the drug therapy.

She went off the hormone replacement therapy and began weekly acupuncture and daily Chinese herbs. After a couple of weeks, Julia found that the herbs actually controlled her moods better than the hormone replacement therapy had. Within two months her hot flashes were also under control. She reported six months later that she felt better than she had in ten years.

As Harriet Beinfield explains, the Kidney system harbors the *jing* energy or essence of the body. *Jing* diminishes naturally with age, as what is used up tends not to be replenished. The diminishing of *jing* is what allows the hormonal imbalances to take place that cause the symptoms of menopause. In a sense herbs can combat the natural effects of aging by replenishing the Kidney essence.

strong in describing what acupuncture *does*, this does not tell us how acupuncture works. From the more traditional view of Chinese medical theory, of course, this is because what really matters is how the technique influences *chi*, something Western science does not yet have the tools to study.

Treating Specific Diseases. The world literature on acupuncture contains thousands of clinical studies of virtually all kinds of illness. Most are published in hundreds of medical journals in the Orient. Again, however, few apply strict Western principles of research design. On this basis, some reviewers of the research state that claims of effectiveness in treating specific ailments are not based on well-performed clinical trials.[39,40]

Critics notwithstanding, the sheer volume of studies from around the world suggests that acupuncture can serve as either a primary or adjunctive treatment for many problems of internal medicine and surgery. For example, recent studies have found beneficial effects for such diverse conditions as tension headache,[41,42] low back pain and tooth extraction,[43] nausea,[44,45] angina pectoris,[46,47,48] osteoarthritis,[49] senile dementia,[50] cervical maturation in pregnancy,[51] migraine,[52] salivary insufficiency,[53] primary dysmenorrhea,[54] and many other ailments.

One study of fifty patients with chronic low back pain (which the American Medical Association considered well designed [55]) found acupuncture to be an effective treatment on a short-term basis.[56] A review of several studies led two researchers to conclude: "Taken together, the results from controlled studies with back pain suggest that a majority (of patients) will derive clinically significant short-term benefits from acupuncture."[57]

Substance Abuse. Another apparently fruitful application is in alcoholism. A controlled study with fifty-four hard-core alcoholic recidivists found acupuncture treatment to bring significant reductions in expressed need for alcohol, drinking episodes, and detox admissions.[58,59]

The U.S. Department of Justice is now exploring the use of acupuncture in the treatment of prisoners who are addicted to alcohol or other drugs. Dr. Michael Smith of the Department of Psychiatry, Lincoln Hospital, The Bronx, New York, is using acupuncture in a probation program for drug abusers. The program is designed to control withdrawal symptoms and craving and to reduce the fears and hostilities that usually accompany drug abuse treatment settings. The program has been so successful it is being replicated in three hundred other locations in the United States and around the world.[60]

Cost-Effectiveness. There is some interesting evidence of the cost-effectiveness in conventional medical practice. Insurance statistics in France show that physicians who practice acupuncture at least half-time use considerably less laboratory examination, hospitalization, and prescriptions for medication.[61] Also, a study in a managed care setting in the United States found patients receiving acupuncture had a reduction in total clinic visits and telephone consultations as well as reduced laboratory, hospitalization, and prescription costs.[62]

STRENGTHS AND LIMITATIONS

As a form of primary care Chinese medicine does well in certain acute conditions such as colds, flu, allergy, and headache. It also has success in treatment of many chronic illnesses with which modern medicine often does not deal successfully. Conditions whose disease process is not clearly understood in allopathic terms may be readily addressed by this tradition.

Many people have experienced the frustration of being told, "Your lab tests are all normal, so there must not be anything wrong with you." Or worse yet, "The feeling you have that something is wrong must be psychosomatic. Go home and rest or get some therapy."

Such is often the case with people suffering from the modern enigmas of chronic fatigue immune dysfunction syndrome (also called chronic fatigue syndrome), environmental illness, fibromyalgia, food sensitivities, and other poorly understood conditions. In Chinese medicine, everything experienced by the patient has meaning and fits into an overall diagnostic picture.

It can also be used to supplement allopathic care, for instance,

Heather

Heather, a thirty-six-year-old college professor, had a thirteen-year history of seasonal allergies with sneezing, itchy eyes, and a great deal of nasal discharge. She had tried multiple medications but they were not working for her. She also suffered from painful menstrual cramps.

She was given a series of eight weekly acupuncture treatments. In addition she was helped to modify her diet, which included avoidance of dairy products, eating regular meals at regular times, and avoiding cold food.

After the fourth treatment she reported her allergies were 90 percent better. Because the treatments were directed not only toward her nose but to the underlying imbalance in her organ network, her menstrual cramps also diminished over the next few months. In the following allergy season she did not need to be treated. Two years later she returned for two treatments and she has been symptom-free for three years.

According to David Field, N.D., L.Ac., "This was a matter of balancing the energy in the body. Heather had a Damp Heat condition, which was caused by a weakness in her Liver. She was expressing this Heat through her eyes and her nose. The drainage of fluid was the way that the body was trying to deal with the accumulation of Damp Heat. The treatment drained the Dampness and the Heat."

in speeding recovery from surgery or, as we saw earlier, as an adjunct to chemotherapy or radiation in cancer treatment.

In 1979 the World Health Organization assembled a list of illnesses that lend themselves to acupuncture treatment.[63] The list is based both on research and clinical experience worldwide. The major illnesses in each of the following categories are included: upper respiratory tract; respiratory system; disorders of the eye; disorders of the mouth, throat, and teeth; gastrointestinal disorders; neurological and musculoskeletal disorders.

More recently, the American Foundation of Medical Acupuncture conducted a review of world clinical literature. Their list of the most frequent successful applications of acupuncture includes the following:

Pain (chronic, surgical, arthritic, malignant, headache, backache, extremity, dental)

Organic lesions (cardiovascular, respiratory, gastrointestinal, skin, urological)

Neurological (peripheral and central)

Substance abuse (drugs, nicotine, food, alcohol)

Gynecological

Psychiatric (depression, anxiety)[64]

This tradition's diagnostic procedures are a unique strength because they allow detection of much more subtle dimensions of health and illness than allopathy is able to address. The practitioner can recognize and intervene in disorders or dysfunction, according to Helms, *"prior to the manifestation of that disorder in a dense histological [physical tissue] form."*[65] It is in this sense that David Walker states: "Chinese medicine is at its *best* as preventive medicine."[66]

A standard part of every training program is recognition of the limitations of the tradition and when to refer the patient elsewhere. Demonstration of this knowledge is also an important part of legal certification and licensing requirements. The most obvious limitations are surgery, emergency medicine (e.g. bone setting), and trauma care, which are the strengths of allopathy.

THE PRACTITIONER-PATIENT RELATIONSHIP

Practitioners cover a wide spectrum in how they view their relationship with the patient. Some of these differences represent the influence of their training and some are a matter of individual personalities.

In classical or Five Element acupuncture, the practitioner may spend the entire treatment session at the patient's side, continuously monitoring the effects of the needling with pulse diagnosis, changing needle positions, perhaps adding moxibustion, and asking the patient for feedback. Essentially, this means almost continuous touch contact in one form or another. This can be felt as a very intimate, interactive process.

At the other extreme are practitioners who work in a more mechanical way—a quick insertion of needles followed by leaving the patient alone in the treatment room, perhaps for a half hour or more. This is a very different experience in terms of the relationship and sense of interpersonal involvement with the practitioner.

Some patients desire a sense of therapeutic relationship more than others. Indeed, some training programs stress that the practitioner is like an energy field the patient enters that provides an energetic context potentiating the treatment; that the emotional and spiritual state of the practitioner has a direct impact on the patient; and that this will significantly influence how the patient responds. Some practitioners even meditate or pray before a session, or may view the treatment process itself as a form of meditation.

Nevertheless, there are also practitioners who are convinced that the needles and herbal treatments are so powerful that a personal, caring relationship is not a major part of the healing equation.

Marie

Marie was a thirty-year-old woman who had suffered a constant, deep chest pain for over a year. Her husband was a physician and she had had dozens of tests looking for heart irregularities, with no positive finding. Her pain was permanently gone after one acupuncture treatment.

According to Dan Kenner, L.Ac., "A lot of people with chest pain have a compression in the rib cage, and if you release it, then the pain is gone. She had neuromuscular tension stored up in the musculature surrounding the rib cage. The acupuncture served to release the tension by loosening the contraction in the muscles, balancing the nervous system, and improving circulation."

EVALUATING PERSONAL RESULTS

There are three ways in which progress is monitored. First is the patient's subjective appraisal of his or her symptoms from treatment to treatment. Second is the practitioner's ongoing diagnostic process, mainly with pulse diagnosis and other forms of observation, at each session, and in some cases as the session progresses. Third are objective tests such as laboratory reports, which may be made available from a regular medical lab. The latter can be a welcome contribution but are not a mainstay of Chinese medicine.

Practitioners' observations are considered relatively objective, but clearly there is a subjective component. Two practitioners may read a person's pulse slightly differently. What is more important is the relativeness from session to session, the changes or patterns observed over time. Hence, even though two practitioners may perceive a different baseline for a certain quality of the pulse, they should observe the same *pattern* of change with time. According to Joseph Helms, M.D., the reading of the pulse is subjective, but it is "objectified" by having the same practitioner, with his or her consistent style, sensing the information over time.

Most practitioners record notes on the qualities of the pulse from session to session and in this way are able to monitor change.

RELATIONSHIP TO OTHER FORMS OF MEDICINE

Chinese medicine does not view itself as exclusive of any other form of medicine. For many ailments it works well on its own, but it also can support or complement other forms of treatment. Its limitations with respect to surgery and emergency medicine were mentioned earlier, but even in these cases it can serve an important supportive role.

Many people use Chinese medicine alongside conventional Western medicine with good results. As discussed earlier, it has shown important benefits in combination with radiation and chemotherapy, including reducing side effects. In pain control acupuncture has been found to enhance and be enhanced by certain allopathic drugs.

Chinese medicine is often combined with other traditions. Medical acupuncturists of course are also trained in allopathy or osteopathy. Many chiropractors are trained in acupuncture as well, and Chinese medicine is a specialty of many naturopaths who use it along with other forms of natural medicine.

COSTS

This tradition tends to be a great deal less expensive than allopathy because it does not involve modern laboratory testing, high-technology equipment, pharmaceuticals, or high malpractice insurance costs. Patient fees are basically for treatment time in the practitioner's office and herbal remedies for those practitioners who use herbs.

The initial session is generally longer and more expensive than subsequent treatments. Initial sessions with nonphysician practitioners may range from $50 to $100 (more for physicians) and follow-up sessions are usually less. The number of sessions varies depending on the nature of the ailment. A typical course of acupuncture treatment may be once or twice a week for a few weeks, with treatments being spaced further apart as time progresses. More difficult chronic illnesses may require treatment over several months. The cost of herbs varies widely, ranging anywhere from $10 to $50 per month.

Insurance Coverage

Insurance companies differ in their coverage, and these differences are influenced by a variety of factors including state regulations, licensure of the provider, and whether medical supervision is required. Some states authorize Medicaid to pay for alcohol and drug abuse treatment by licensed or certified acupuncturists. In addition, some states mandate general insurance coverage for acupuncture treatment. Because of the rapidly changing regulatory climate in the field of health care, you need to inquire about current coverage in your state.

Janet

Janet, a woman in her early forties, had low back pain and ulcerative colitis. One morning she noticed blood in her stool. In previous episodes she had gone to the hospital, but based on her experience there she decided to call her acupuncturist first.

According to Dan Kenner, L.Ac., "In cases like this, one treatment can often stop the crisis. There are two points associated with the large intestine on both sides of the fifth lumbar on the back. Through pulse diagnosis, palpation, and by manipulating the needle, I found that these points were blocked. After they opened up there was immediate relief of the low back pain and intestinal cramping. With one treatment the bleeding stopped and did not start again.

"Acupuncture could be considered an excellent treatment for any stress-related disorder, and ulcerative colitis has a high stress component. Because of the extreme sensitivity of the nerve endings in the gastrointestinal mucosa, people under severe stress often have an overstimulation that results in erosion of mucous membranes, bleeding, and copious mucus discharge.

"The treatment caused a release of *chi* that had congested or stagnated in the large intestine. People often somaticize their emotional stress, and where they do it depends on their individual typology. For her it was in the large intestine, whereas the next person might have heart palpitations or panic disorder."

CHOOSING A PRACTITIONER

Although acupuncture and herbology are different kinds of treatment, most credentialing bodies consider the use of Chinese herbs as part of acupuncture practice.

State Regulation

States vary in who they allow to practice acupuncture. At this writing, twenty-two states license, certify, or register acupuncturists: [67]

Alaska	Massachusetts	Rhode Island
California	Montana	Texas
Colorado	Nevada	Utah
District of Columbia	New Jersey	Vermont
Florida	New Mexico	Virginia
Hawaii	North Carolina	Washington
Iowa	Oregon	Wisconsin
Maine		

In Alabama and Illinois, the practice of acupuncture is limited to M.D.s, D.O.s, and D.C.s. In the following twelve other states it is limited to M.D.s and D.O.s:

Arizona	Louisiana	New Hampshire
Georgia	Minnesota	North Dakota
Indiana	Mississippi	Ohio
Kentucky	Nebraska	West Virginia

The following states allow acupuncture under the supervision of a licensed physician:

Connecticut	Michigan	Pennsylvania
Delaware	Missouri	South Carolina
Kansas	New York	

There are no regulations on acupuncture in the following states:

Arkansas	Oklahoma
Idaho	South Dakota
Maryland	Wyoming

Physician or Nonphysician?

Some medical acupuncturists tend to refer to nonphysician practitioners of acupuncture as lay acupuncturists and take the position that acupuncture is the practice of medicine and should only be done by licensed physicians. They also hold that one should not have acupuncture until there has been a medical diagnosis by a physician, and that such practice should only be used with medical supervision. The concern, of course, is over the risk of an undiagnosed or misdiagnosed disease progressing to an incurable stage.

Many nonphysicians take the perspective that medical acupuncturists' primary training is in Western rather than Chinese medicine, and as a result, most lack sufficient hours of acupuncture education and training to be fully competent with this highly specialized method. Schools of Chinese medicine usually involve three to four years of study.

Some people feel more confident being treated by a Western-trained physician who can combine aspects of the two traditions. There can also be advantages to this in terms of insurance coverage. Other people seek a practitioner who is more thoroughly committed to and grounded in the broader philosophy and practice of Chinese medicine.

Peak Performance

In the fall of 1993, the sports world was shaken when a small group of Chinese female runners obliterated several long-standing world records in a span of six days. This sudden meteoric rise into international prominence by the Chinese women immediately gave rise to suspicions of drug use, which were unproven. Making the accomplishments even more unbelievable was the fact that many of the records broken had been set years before by Eastern European women now known to have used illegal performance-enhancing drugs liberally in their training.

Affronted by the suspicions, the Chinese sports authorities shared their secret: a rigorous training program and a special diet that included traditional Chinese herbs and a mineral-rich potion made from the *dong chong xia cao* worm. World records are usually broken by mere tenths of seconds or a few seconds, and experts agree that it is unlikely that the sheer magnitude of the improvement on the old records could be attributable to hard training alone. This may be the most dramatic and visible evidence yet of the powerful effects Chinese herbs can have on the body.

Organizations

The National Commission for Certification of Acupuncturists (NCCA) was chartered in 1984 to promote nationally recognized standards for safe and competent acupuncture practice. The NCCA conducts a certification exam with both written and practical portions, including clean needle techniques. Practitioners who are certified are designated "Diplomate in Acupuncture" or "Dipl.Ac. (NCCA)," and are listed in the annual *Directory of National Board Certified Acupuncturists.*

Ninety percent of the states that license acupuncturists recognize NCCA certification or use the NCCA exam in their licensing process. This is a good credential to ask about, though *it is unnecessary if the practitioner is otherwise licensed or certified by the state.* Some insurance companies use NCCA certification as a criterion for reimbursement.

At this writing the NCCA is in the process of developing an exam to certify competence in herbalism separately from the practice of acupuncture. It is possible that such an exam may be presented to state legislatures to regulate the practice of herbalism by practitioners who do not use acupuncture. Address: 1424 16th St. N.W., Suite 501, Washington, DC 20036, phone (202) 232–1404, FAX (202) 462–6157.

The American Association of Acupuncture and Oriental Medicine (AAAOM), founded in 1981, is the largest membership organization for practitioners, with over 1600 members. It promotes public education about acupuncture and advocacy for the profession. An individual member in AAAOM is someone who has achieved diplomate status with the NCCA or is licensed by a state using equivalent criteria. Address: 433 Front St., Catasaugua, PA 18032, phone (610) 266–1433, FAX (610) 264–2768.

The National Accreditation Commission for Schools and Colleges of Acupuncture and Oriental Medicine (NACSCAOM). Another criterion, though less important, and one that applies to *non*physician practitioners is whether they have graduated from a program accredited by NACSCAOM. About half the current schools have this status, but many perfectly fine programs do not, as it is not a requirement in the field. Address: 8403 Colesville Rd., Suite 370, Silver Spring, MD 20910, phone (301) 608–9680, FAX (301) 608–9576.

The American Academy of Medical Acupuncture (AAMA) was formed in 1987 to represent the education and practice interests of well-trained physician acupuncturists. It restricts its membership to physicians (M.D.s and D.O.s). Currently it has

Sue

Sue had been suffering from frequent anxiety attacks accompanied by rapid heartbeat, dryness of the mouth, restlessness, and insomnia. Though she was using psychotherapy, she felt it had been insufficient for her needs.

In the oriental tradition such cases are often what are called *shen* disturbances, disorders affecting a person's spirit or soul.

Chronically anxious patients are often exhausted but unable to relax. A state of deep relaxation is often an immediate benefit of treatment, but the longer lasting benefits are a general reduction of nervousness and a reexperiencing of a sense of ease and well-being.

Dan Kenner, L.Ac., an acupuncturist in Santa Rosa, California, describes the process: "Sue slept deeply during the treatments and I allowed her to rest for a time after I was finished because the changes in her respiration, pulse, and demeanor were so profound.

"After a course of eight treatments she reported that her psychotherapy was going extremely well and that her therapist was amazed at how quickly she was moving through issues with which she had struggled for years.

"Acupuncture can release unconscious holding of tension as the patient enters a state of deep relaxation. During this process, unconscious emotional issues may surface as well. I often suggest that patients carefully observe moods, dreams, or unusual mental states that may occur within a couple of days following treatment. These states may be part of a healing process of emotional or psychological catharsis."

eight hundred members. Since any licensed physician is allowed to practice acupuncture regardless of training or competency, membership in the AAMA is a good guideline as to preparation.

Full members have a minimum of 220 hours of formal training or the equivalent in an apprenticeship program acceptable to the AAMA, two years experience practicing medical acupuncture, and a personal endorsement by an academy member. Associate members meet part but not all of these requirements. A proficiency exam has been established and a board certification process has been created. Address: 5820 Wilshire Blvd., Suite 500, Los Angeles, CA 90036, phone (213) 937–5514, FAX (213) 937–0959.

Conclusion

Ultimately, your choice of a practitioner should be based on three points. First, they should meet state legal regulations to practice. Second, you should be familiar enough with their background to know what their professional and philosophical orientation is, and that you feel comfortable with their approach. Third, and most important, you should feel comfortable in their presence and find it easy to trust them. This can be determined both in an initial, exploratory meeting, as well as by feedback or recommendations of friends or others whose judgment you respect.

CHAPTER 3

AYURVEDA: THE WISDOM
OF THE ANCIENTS

"It is the purpose of Ayurveda to give us the means
of health and healing on a physical and psychological
level so that we can pursue the path of Yoga."
　　　　　　　　　　—DAVID FRAWLEY, O.M.D.[1]

More than five thousand years ago a group of holy men known
as the *Rishis* compiled the ancient Hindu philosophical and
spiritual texts called the Vedas. These are a remarkably elabo-
rate system of knowledge, comprising the science of life as revealed to the *Rishis* through what today we might call divine
inspiration.

They comprise four main branches, which are called the Vedic
sciences: Self-knowledge, yoga, Vedic astrology, and Ayurveda.
Ayurveda is the science that deals with physical healing, diet,
herbs, and massage or bodywork. As reflected in Frawley's statement above, it was originally intended as a means to support
the body so that spiritual development could be pursued unhin-
dered by health concerns. The yoga to which he refers is a broad
term roughly meaning "right path." It encompasses all aspects
of living healthfully and harmoniously in the world.

Ralph

Ralph was a thirty-eight-year-old engineer who had been suffering for two years with Ménière's disease. This involves ringing in the ears, dizziness, and gradual loss of hearing. He was also having marital difficulties, which he attributed in part to the syndrome.

His metabolic type was *pitta-vata*. He was given a combination of herbs and was instructed in *nasya*, which involves placing sesame oil in each nostril and inhaling to draw the oil up into the sinuses. He also put the oil in his ears, used sesame oil massage, aromatherapy, and *pranayama* (alternate nostril breathing).

Within three months his symptoms were gone and test results showed his hearing was improving. Shortly thereafter his wife became pregnant. Treatment lasted three months.

As a result of westerners' desire to discover alternative medical traditions, the spiritual context of Ayurvedic teachings has often been sidestepped in the interest of finding remedies for modern ailments. This narrower view has not been resisted by the modern Ayurveda teachers, since it has thrust Ayurveda into the public eye and stimulated a great deal of interest. Still, to think of Ayurveda only as medicine narrows the focus considerably from its original purposes.

The proponents of Ayurveda claim it to be the oldest system of natural healing on earth and the common root of many of today's other medical traditions. Its methods are noninvasive, nontoxic, and heavily dependent on the individual's willingness to participate voluntarily in a healthier way of life.

This is the traditional health care approach of India involving the eight principal branches of medicine: pediatrics, gynecology, obstetrics, ophthalmology, geriatrics, otolaryngology (ear, nose, and throat), general medicine, and surgery. Today it is used by 80 percent of the population, although it exists side by side with modern allopathy. Entire hospitals and more than a quarter of a million practitioners promote this tradition.

Ayurveda's rapidly growing identity as an alternative medical tradition in the United States has been led by the mercurial success of Deepak Chopra, M.D., an endocrinologist and former chief of staff of New England Memorial Hospital in Stoneham, Massachusetts. A charismatic speaker and the author of several best-selling books, Dr. Chopra has helped bring Ayurveda to the forefront of alternative medicine in a very brief period of time. He was instrumental in the development of the Center for Mind/Body Medicine in La Jolla, California, which trains health care professionals in state-of-the-art treatment programs.

While Ayurveda has the smallest number of practitioners of any medical tradition in this country, those numbers are expanding, with a proliferation of training programs. Part of Chopra's vision is for Ayurveda to become a routine part of mainstream medical education.[2]

KEY PRINCIPLES

The Vital Energy: Prana

Like other traditions of nature-based medicine, Ayurveda is built upon a concept of vital energy. Called *prana*, it is the primal energy that enlivens the body and mind. Analogous to the Chinese concept of *chi*, it is the unseen power that is the basis of all life and healing. Since it is considered to have the qualities of a nutrient that can be taken into the body through the breath, breathing exercises hold an important role in health promotion according to Ayurveda. The breath is a direct way to draw in and build life energy within oneself. Ayurveda uses a variety of breathing exercises called *pranayama* for imbibing *prana* and using it to enliven the body and promote healing.

The Five Elements

At the heart of Ayurveda is the concept that all of existence comprises five basic principles or elements: earth, air, fire, water, and ether. More than their literal meanings, these terms represent principles of action and interaction that guide and shape all that exists on the material plane and in life processes. To illustrate the workings of these principles, Ayurvedic physician Dr. Vasant Lad offers the following example:

> The solid state of water, ice, is a manifestation of the Earth principle. Latent heat (Fire) in the ice liquefies it, manifesting the Water principle; and then eventually it turns into steam, expressing the Air principle. The steam disappears into Ether, or space. Thus the five basic elements, Ether, Air, Fire, Water, and Earth, are present in one substance. All five originated in the energy issuing from Cosmic Consciousness; all five are present in all matter in the universe. Thus, energy and matter are one.[3]

The actions and interactions of these five elements serve as the basis for understanding health, illness, individual constitution, and how to restore and maintain harmony in the body.

Individual Constitution

At conception, each of us is endowed with a certain constitution that is ours for life. This constitution is our unique pattern for

Jonathan

A thirty-seven-year-old pharmacist, Jonathan sought Ayurveda for gallstones and clinical depression. He was taking conventional medicines for both conditions, including antidepressants, and was experiencing loose bowels three to four times per day, weight loss, and frequent outbursts of anger. He also had a skin rash as a drug side effect. His symptoms had continued for two months.

Upon examination he was determined to be *pitta* predominant and *vata* secondary. A treatment plan was devised to pacify both *pitta* and *vata*. A *panchakarma* detoxification regime was prescribed once a week for four weeks. He also undertook a daily program of relaxation and focusing similar to meditation.

The *panchakarma* consisted of *snehan* (an herbal oil massage with a focus on specific *marma* points), an herbal decoction sauna (herbs placed in the sauna so their vapors could be inhaled), other aromatherapy, herb tea, and music therapy. He also took an *amlaki* compound as a nutritional supplement, another herbal formula called *suta*, and one called *shant*.

Within six weeks he reported that his gallbladder symptoms, rash, and angry outbursts had all ceased and he was off all his other medications. He completed the treatment two weeks later.

As Dr. Shanbhag explains, when a person is under stress the metabolism of the liver and gallbladder go out of balance. These problems are considered related to *pitta* metabolism since it is responsible for digestion. The herbs rebalanced *pitta*, thus improving liver and gallbladder metabolism so that the stones could be dissolved or passed. Dr. Shanbhag considered the emotional problems a *vata* imbalance, which was corrected with the help of the *shant* and the integrated relaxation and focusing.

how the five elements are organized within us and how they manifest in our life.

In our body the five elements undergo a further step of organization into three broader principles or elements known as the *doshas*: *vata* (ether and air), *pitta* (fire and water), and *kapha* (earth and water). Collectively, the three *doshas* are organized into our *tridosha*. They are considered the basic constituents that govern our physiological and psychological functions. In fact, together they determine our personal metabolism and our psychophysiological or mind/body type. The unique pattern that they take in each of us at our conception is called our *prakriti*.

There are seven general patterns of *prakriti* that are possible, with many subtle variations. The *prakriti* for each person is diagnosed and described according to which *doshas* naturally predominate and which are least influential in that person's functioning.

Some people have a *prakriti* in which there is a clear dominance of a single *dosha*—either *vata*, *pitta*, or *kapha*. Others have a slightly more complex *prakriti* in which there are equal influences of multiple doshas, such as *vata-pitta*, *pitta-kapha*, *vata-kapha*, and the most complex, *vata-pitta-kapha*. The influences and qualities of the individual *doshas* are briefly described below.[4]

Vata. Representing the elements air and ether, *vata* is the lightest of the *doshas*. As such, it represents easy movement at all levels and in all ways. *Vata* governs the movement of cells circulating in the body, the movement of fluids and materials through the cells and through the body, the activity of organs and muscles as they perform their functions, the motor and sensory functions of the person as they move through the world, and the movement of thoughts through the mind.

People in whom vata predominates tend to be active, alert, and restless. They need to be involved in movement and activity in order to feel in a state of harmony. They usually have a lot of energy, though they may not be doing anything with it. They are often fiddling, doodling, and moving around. They tend to disperse or sometimes waste energy. In the same way, *vata* people are more likely to disperse their money easily. They may fritter it away at a flea market and may even dispense with a large inheritance rather quickly. A *vata* person may prefer to be an artist or musician rather than an employee of someone else. *Vata disperses.*

Pitta. *Pitta* is often described as transformative energy. The digestion and transformation of food into energy, and ultimately into the tissues of the body, is considered a *pitta* function. *Pitta* governs the digestive functions, body temperature, and other metabolic functions. Fire is a good symbol to represent this *dosha.*

Pitta people are often involved in transformative kinds of activity, taking one thing and changing it into something else. They may also have fiery qualities in their personality, such as a lot of anger, irritability, a red face, aggressiveness, or competitiveness. *Pitta* people would be more inclined to budget their money and transform it into useful things or projects to improve their standard of living. They make good CEOs. *Pitta transforms.*

Kapha. *Kapha* is the densest element, providing the physical structure and contents of the body. Comprised of earth and water, it represents accumulation and the formation of dense structure. *Kapha* heals wounds, fills spaces, and brings physical strength and resiliency to the body. *Kapha* is bodily tissue, fluid, and substance.

Kapha people tend to be heavier, slower moving, more solid, and have greater muscular strength. They may also be more stable and grounded, with a more steady, tranquil personality. They would tend to hold onto money and would be more likely to be wealthy because of their tendency to accumulate. *Kapha* people don't like to move around much and they tend to make good middle managers. *Kapha accumulates.*

Health and Illness

In Ayurveda, health is a state of balance and harmony among all of these forces within the person and between the person and their surroundings. The optimal state is one in which the person is living in accordance with their *prakriti* at conception. In other words, their lifestyle and current state of health reflect a perfect alignment with their unique constitution.

Illness occurs when the person falls out of equilibrium with this inborn pattern. Imbalances in specific *doshas* can be caused by chronic stress, eating certain foods, inadequate rest, environmental toxins, and many other factors. And, in keeping with Ayurveda's focus on mind/body relations, repressed emotions are considered an important cause for imbalance. For example, repressed fear causes imbalance in *vata*, anger will cause excess *pitta*, and envy, greed, and attachment will aggravate *kapha*.

An imbalance can be comprised of either an excess or a deficiency of *vata*, *pitta*, or *kapha* beyond what is optimal for the individual. The new dysfunctional configuration or pattern that arises is called one's *vikriti*, which literally means "deviating from nature."

For example, a person's *prakriti* may have *pitta* as the dominant *dosha*, but such aggravating influences as cold weather, dry or moving air, repressed fear, or lack of rest may result in *pitta* being overtaken by *vata*. Thus their *vikriti* shows *vata* as the predominant *dosha*.

The resulting state of disharmony will weaken their *agni*, the fire that governs their metabolism, leading to a state of lowered resistance and the buildup of toxins in the body. Such toxins are called *ama*. They are circulated throughout the body and build up in certain locations, causing symptoms and ultimately disease.

Types of Disease. Diseases are classified according to whether their origins are psychological, spiritual, or physical; where they manifest in the body; and what *dosha* they represent. Since we each have all three *doshas*, we can have disorders caused by

Claudine

Claudine, a thirty-three-year-old secretary, had chronic acne on her face, neck, and shoulders. Her appearance was of particular concern to her in her work as it involved making frequent presentations to groups of people. The acne was inflamed with a red base. She had been treated with all the conventional dermatological treatments including tetracycline and other antibiotics as well as steroid injections in her acne. She would routinely get steroid injections for quick results prior to a presentation.

In her first visit to the Ayurvedic practitioner it was determined that she seemed to be following a healthy lifestyle and her body type is *pitta* predominant. She was put on a *pitta*-pacifying diet.

Claudine was given *shankha bhasma* three times daily and another herbal formula called *champa* for balancing the female hormonal system. She took the formulas for ten weeks, accompanied by a relaxation and focusing program. After ten weeks she reported that the acne had completely subsided on her face and diminished on her shoulders and she had not had to take any steroid injections.

She was instructed to change clothing, shampoo, and soaps to which she might be sensitive and to maintain the diet and herbal formulas to continue the progress on her shoulders.

According to Dr. Shanbhag, the *shankha bhasma* worked by balancing the *pitta* metabolism and the *champa* served to rebalance the female hormonal system, an imbalance of which is considered one of the causative factors of acne.

imbalances in any one or all of them. However, we most commonly have problems associated with our predominant *dosha*. For example, according to Dr. Lad, people with the *vata* constitution are more likely to have *vata* conditions such as intestinal gas, lower back pain, sciatica, arthritis, paralysis, neuralgia, and nervous system diseases.

Pitta people are more likely to have gallbladder, liver and bile disorders, hyperacidity, peptic ulcer, gastritis, inflammatory diseases, and skin disorders such as hives and rash.

Kapha people are more likely to have *kapha* diseases such as tonsillitis, bronchitis, sinusitis, and lung congestion.

People can have diseases that do not necessarily correspond with their predominant *dosha*. As explained by Janhavi Morton, a practitioner in Santa Rosa, California, "Anyone, even a *kapha* or *vata*, can have a *pitta* disease, but luckily they will be able to get rid of it more quickly because *pitta* is not their primary constitution. A *pitta* has a harder time bringing an inflammatory *pitta* disease under control because their very nature is hot, and therefore disposed toward *pitta* conditions."[5]

Food and the Six Tastes. The dietary therapy of Ayurveda is oriented toward rebalancing the *doshas*. Thus, there are specific diets for reducing or "pacifying" each *dosha*, depending on which one is out of balance.

The tastes of food are a key in Ayurveda because they provide important clues as to which foods are helpful and which are harmful in balancing one's *tridosha*. The six tastes and examples are:

- Sweet (sugar, milk, butter, rice, breads, pasta)
- Sour (yogurt, lemon, cheese)
- Salty (salt)
- Pungent (spicy foods, ginger, hot peppers, cumin)
- Bitter (green leafy vegetables, turmeric)
- Astringent (beans, lentils, pomegranate)

According to Dr. Mary Jo Cravatta, a practitioner in Palo Alto, California, "Everyone should have all six tastes at their main meal but in different proportions, depending upon what *dosha* they need to balance."[6]

When we have a preference (but not a strong craving) for certain tastes, this usually indicates that those tastes are needed to balance our predominant *dosha*. On the other hand, extreme cravings or addictions to tastes indicate an underlying imbalance that will be further aggravated by those tastes.

The effects the tastes have on our *doshas* are as follows:

- Sweet, sour, and salty *decrease vata*, and *increase kapha.*
- Pungent, bitter, and astringent *decrease kapha*, and *increase vata.*
- Sweet, bitter, and astringent *decrease pitta.*
- Sour, salty, and pungent *increase pitta.*

The Three Malas. Another important concept is elimination of waste materials from the body. A great deal of attention is given to detoxification and elimination of *ama* through the three *malas*: sweat, urine, and feces. The efficient production and elimination of these are considered absolutely essential to health. The qualities and characteristics of the three *malas* are taken into account in diagnosis and assessment of overall health.

Treatment of Illness

Ayurveda's first priority is prevention, health promotion, and enhancement. However, it also presents a complete system for treating illness. In both cases, the overall goal is to reestablish balance among the *doshas,* and to purify and harmonize the entire mind/body system. Thus, disease entities or pathogens are not the main object of treatment, but rather it is the person's overall integration and the consequent host resistance that are of concern.

Emily

Emily, twenty-four, complained of irregular bowel movements from two to five days apart. Her pulses revealed a body type of *pitta-vata* and an imbalance of *vata*. People who are mostly *pitta* usually have good digestion with one or two bowel movements per day. However, the colon is the seat of *vata*, and constipation or irregularity is an expression of *vata* excess in the colon. She also had irregular menstrual periods and PMS.

Emily was instructed in a *vata*-pacifying diet: warm cooked foods; sour, salty, and smooth creamy sweet tastes; no raw vegetables; no light or dry foods like popcorn or corn chips. She was also given some herbs and was instructed in daily sesame oil massage. All these guidelines were designed to calm her *vata*.

She returned in a month for another consultation and reported having a bowel movement daily. By the end of six months her periods were regular and she had no more symptoms of PMS.

Culture and Illness

Ayurveda offers some very interesting insights into why we face the diseases that are so prevalent in modern societies. Because *vata* governs the nervous system, it is the *dosha* that is most easily thrown out of balance by chronic stress. The hectic, fast-paced lifestyle that many follow in Western society thus contributes to *vata* imbalances on a mass scale. Fast food, fast cars, commuting, tight schedules, and other pressures to think and move quickly foster a culturewide state of *vata* imbalance, which has become the norm.

One consequence is that this translates into dietary behavior on a mass scale involving craving of sweet, sour, and salty tastes. These tastes accompany foods that, if consumed in inordinate quantities, bring the predictably negative health effects of excess sugar, fat, and salt intake.

Another consequence is that *vata* imbalance can lead to chronic fatigue, which can allow deterioration of the integrity of vital bodily systems. This may be a factor in chronic fatigue immune dysfunction syndrome (CFIDS), in which the immune system is stuck in a hyperactive state. The immune system itself seems to be in a perpetual state of *vata* imbalance and churns out inordinately high levels of hormones that have toxic effects on the body, causing a wide variety of symptoms.[7]

According to Ayurveda, one of the most effective antidotes for *vata* imbalance is meditation. And, indeed, much research on the medical effects of meditation has shown significant health benefits for immune-related and stress-related illnesses as well as many other conditions. The fact that Ayurveda so strongly encourages meditation makes it an especially appropriate tradition for many of modern society's ills.

VARIATIONS WITHIN THE TRADITION

In the West there are two major currents of training and practice in Ayurveda. The first is offered by a diverse variety of teachers and practitioners, many of whom are either from India or were trained there. Though some of these are licensed as primary health care providers in this country, many are not, and instead function in the role of health consultant or health educator.

There is no organization connecting them and many work as free spirits, offering varying degrees of consultation or training. Best-known among them are Deepak Chopra, M.D., associated with the Center for Mind/Body Medicine in La Jolla, California; former Indian medical school professor Dr. Vasant Lad of the Ayurvedic Institute in Albuquerque, New Mexico; and Dr. David Frawley of the American Institute of Vedic Studies in Santa Fe. All three have written popular books about Ayurveda. Other leading proponents include Dr. Vivek Shanbhag of the department of Ayurvedic medicine at Bastyr University of Natural Health Sciences, Seattle, and Dr. Virender Sodhi of the American School of Ayurvedic Sciences in Bellevue, Washington.

The other major current is led by devotees of Maharishi Mahesh Yogi, the Indian spiritual teacher who introduced transcendental meditation (TM) to the West. In 1980 this group coined the term "Maharishi Ayur-Ved," which incorporates TM as part of an Ayurvedic approach.

This group is highly organized and offers training programs to licensed health care providers at Maharishi International University (MIU) in Fairfield, Iowa, and at other centers around the country.

In 1993 MIU created its College of Maharishi Ayur-Ved to offer degree- and non-degree-granting courses of study. According to Stuart Rothenberg, M.D., codean of the college, one of its goals is to establish Ayurveda as a recognized medical discipline in the United States by structuring a professional academic curriculum of study beginning at the undergraduate level and culminating with a doctoral level degree in clinical Ayurveda, comparable in stature to the M.D., D.O., D.C., N.D., and so on.

Maharishi Ayur-Ved's emphasis on meditation is consistent with the view of Ayurveda as a complete science of mind/body relations. In fact, according to Rothenberg, the development of consciousness is really the linchpin of this tradition. The historic emphasis on this aspect has eroded over the centuries, to the point where today the majority of practitioners in India practice much the same way as Western allopathic physicians, prescribing substances more as physical medicine.

Rothenberg says, "While that has its place in Ayurvedic medicine, without the science of consciousness and the technologies to develop consciousness, the heart of Ayurveda is missing."[8]

Nicholas

Nicholas was in his early thirties. He had been over-weight his entire life and complained of feeling very sluggish and unmotivated. He had a habit of sleeping late, could not get himself to exercise, would overeat and then feel uncomfortable afterward, and had a lot of sinus congestion and mucus.

Kapha and *pitta* were equally predominant and both were imbalanced. Since these are both balanced by bitter and astringent tastes he was instructed to eat more dark green leafy vegetables, beans, cabbage, broccoli, cauliflower, and apples and eliminate heavy or oily foods, particularly cheeses and meats.

He was to eat his main meal at noon since this is a *pitta* period and *pitta* makes for stronger digestion. He was also to eat more lightly at night and go to bed by ten. His mood and motivation gradually improved and he lost thirty pounds in six months.

According to Dr. Cravatta, his *dosha* was balanced by altering his eating patterns to be more in harmony with the metabolic cycles of the day. If one eats a heavy meal during *kapha* time (evenings) it is less likely to be fully metabolized and more likely to contribute to weight gain. Thus for Nicholas it was necessary to eat as early and as lightly as possible.

He also needed to go to bed by ten so that he could wake up earlier in the morning. The later one wakes up during the morning *kapha* period (6:00 to 10:00 A.M.) the more sluggish one will feel. Thus his overall improvement was attributed to his change of diet and his coming into harmony with the natural metabolic cycles of the day.

Maharishi Ayur-Ved thus presents itself as a way of returning to the original classical principles by treating consciousness as a central issue in health, along with the other aspects of Ayurveda such as herbs, diet, other forms of treatment, exercise, and lifestyle.

Other Ayurveda practitioners agree that consciousness plays a key role in health and also recommend meditation. They point out, however, that TM is only one of many forms of meditation that can support the goals and principles of Ayurveda.

Both groups would agree that meditation should not be imposed upon people who are not open to it and who are seeking a more Western model of medical treatment. Hence, both varieties of practitioners avoid expectations or demands that patients pursue meditation and are happy to treat people who have no interest in it. The Maharishi practitioners have a well-organized and widely available approach, which they hold to be superior to other forms of meditation, to recommend for those who are receptive to it.

Another difference between the two kinds of practitioners is that proponents of the Maharishi approach have their own brand of herbal formulas, some of which have undergone scientific study in university research. There are over 150 companies in India that also produce traditional Ayurvedic formulas, many of which are available through practitioners or health food stores in the United States. It is difficult to judge the relative effectiveness of different products since there are many possible variations of the formulas and no standard means for comparing them.

PROCEDURES AND TECHNIQUES

Visiting an Ayurvedic practitioner usually involves an extensive individual interview for taking a health history and making a diagnostic assessment. Diagnosis means diagnosing one's constitution (*prakriti* and *vikriti*), not diagnosing specific diseases in Western terms. Once the diagnosis is established, it is followed by detailed dietary guidelines and possibly recommendations for herbs and other treatments.

Diagnostic Methods

Written Questionnaires. Many practitioners use a written questionnaire at the time of intake to establish the person's *tridosha.* This includes questions about the body, metabolism, habits, sleep, self-image, interests, preferences, emotional and psychological attributes, and other aspects that will help to paint an accurate picture of the person's overall characteristics.

Pulse Diagnosis. In pulse diagnosis what the practitioner is feeling are patterns of vibration that represent the metabolic processes happening in the body at that time. Every process that occurs sends out a vibratory signal. In Ayurveda there are three basic pulses on each wrist, corresponding to each of the three *doshas—vata, pitta,* and *kapha.* There are also pulses representing combinations of those and each has several subdivisions.

As Dr. Rothenberg states: "There are many different aspects of physiology that you feel in the pulse. So when we say we're getting to know the person, we're not just talking with them. We're really getting something like an X ray or fingerprint, the patterns of vibration that characterize the person. Each pulse also has several different layers, so we can actually go back in time with the pulse and see what the body was like seven years or seventeen years ago."[9]

Pulse diagnosis is an art that can require many years to develop to its highest potential. Famous Ayurvedic physicians in India have given astonishingly precise diagnoses of diseases and the condition of internal organs, confirmed by modern high-tech diagnostic tests.

Other Methods of Diagnosis. Practitioners also consider the appearance of the tongue, face, lips, nails, and eyes for diagnostic information. Finally, some practitioners use laboratory tests of blood, urine, and stools to assist with diagnosis.

Dietary Guidance

The most basic form of intervention is diet, which must be carefully tailored to the person's unique constitutional type and status. Certain foods are believed to pacify or aggravate certain *doshas.* Since the goal of treatment is to restore proper balance among the *doshas,* foods that will support this rebalancing process are chosen.

Practitioners usually give very specific dietary guidelines, with lists of foods to eat and to avoid. In some cases, a diet may be designed to pacify one *dosha* while not aggravating another. For example, James was suffering from a buildup of toxins in his liver, a *pitta* problem, and was also under a lot of stress. His practitioner recommended a *pitta*-pacifying but not *vata*-aggravating diet as shown below.

Rasayanas

A *rasayana* is a regime you use on a regular basis, of which there are two kinds: herbal *rasayanas* (herbal dietary supplements that help to balance the *doshas*) and behavioral *rasayanas* (individualized behavior or lifestyle changes appropriate to one's *tridosha*).

Herbs. Herbal *rasayanas* have been traditionally recommended for good health and longevity. They include preparations of fruits, herbs, and some minerals; these formulas have no equiva-

Laurel

Laurel was a secretary in her midtwenties who had been struggling with anxiety and panic attacks for a year and a half. She had been on disability for two months and was taking an antidepressant. The anxiety problems were so severe she had to be driven by a friend to her appointment.

Dr. Cravatta found her metabolic type to be *vata-pitta* and she had a *prana vata* imbalance. This is a *vata* imbalance manifested by very fast, scattered mental activity. In Ayurveda, fear and anxiety are considered *vata* emotions; the greater the imbalance, the more fear and anxiety.

Dr. Cravatta explains that although meditation is a natural antidote to *vata* imbalance, people with *prana vata* usually have difficulty meditating. An alternative way to pacify *vata* and calm the mind is slow *pranayama* (alternate nostril breathing).

This recommendation was accompanied by an herbal combination (MA-666) to pacify *vata* and valerian root to calm *prana vata*, taken at night to promote calm and sleep. Sesame oil massage was also part of Laurel's program. She was seen three times and was back at work within two months.

lent counterparts in conventional Western medicine. They may be in many forms including tinctures, teas, compotes (pastes or jellies), pills, or powders that are mixed with food.

The classical Ayurvedic texts prescribe certain *rasayanas* for specific diseases, for promoting general health by increasing resistance to disease, activating tissue repair mechanisms, and arresting or reversing the deterioration of aging. Each *rasayana*

73

may contain ten to twenty separate herbs and each herb may have hundreds or thousands of chemical components.

This is one area where Ayurveda and allopathy differ markedly in the use of medications. According to Ayurvedic thought, by using the combined herbal preparation, which sometimes includes whole plant products, rather than isolated chemicals that we would consider the active ingredients, the various chemical constituents work synergistically, mitigating any harmful side effects.[10]

Yoga Asanas. These are yoga postures that are recommended for purposes of neuromuscular integration. A routine of several postures for ten to twenty minutes each day may be suggested. One popular asana is known as the Sun Salute, which combines stretching, balance, and mild aerobic exercise. Some asanas are given for the specific purpose of stimulating certain organs, depending on one's symptoms or medical condition. Of the varieties of yoga that have been developed, Ayurveda is most aligned with hatha yoga, the yoga of the physical body.[11]

Pranayama. Pranayama involves a set of breathing exercises that have the effects of soothing the nervous system, inducing relaxation, regulating the breathing process, and balancing the hemispheres of the brain. The major technique is alternate nostril breathing, in which you close off one nostril by pressing a finger against it while exhaling and inhaling through the other. Then you switch sides and repeat the process through the other nostril. This alternating process is continued for five minutes or so.

Meditation. One of the key principles of Ayurveda is that disease arises when we do not listen to the body's wisdom. Meditation is thus promoted as a way to listen to the body and for stress reduction and improving general well-being. Originating in India, of course, Ayurveda comes from a cultural context rich with many different traditions of meditation.

The TM technique is advocated among practitioners of Maharishi Ayur-Ved. This involves meditating twice per day for twenty minutes by repeating a mantra. Other forms of meditation may involve other ways of concentrating the mind using a variety of breathing exercises or by chanting.

As will be seen in Chapter 6 on Mind/Body Medicine, meditation has been found to have many beneficial physiological effects by inducing the relaxation response.

Massage

In Ayurveda the geography of the body includes 107 *marma* points (roughly similar in concept to the acupuncture points in Chinese medicine). Ayurvedic massage, called *abhyanga*, includes stimulation of these *marma* points through touch and use of medicinal oils to help in rebalancing the *doshas* and the flow of energy through the body. Massage is also used to help move toxins through the body so they can be eliminated.

Warm sesame oil is sometimes recommended in a daily routine of self-massage in the morning before bathing to help maintain vitality. Sesame oil is capable of many complex physiological interactions that promote health, including anticancer, anti-inflammatory, and antibacterial properties. It is also used as a mouth rinse after toothbrushing for oral hygiene.

Panchakarma

Panchakarma is an intensive detoxification process that takes place over several days, ideally one to two weeks. It may be used once or twice per year to eliminate and prevent the accumulation of *ama* (physiological impurities). Somewhat like a personal health retreat, it involves many different Ayurvedic modalities as well as healthy food, comfort, and deep rest. Its main aim is to promote health and longevity.

Regular procedures include massage (*abhyanga*) with special herbal oils that help the body release toxins that have accumulated in its tissues so they can be eliminated. This may be followed by steam treatments and herbalized enemas (*basti*). Another technique is nasal administration of herbs (*nasya*). One procedure at some centers involves ingestion of large amounts of clarified butter in the early morning on four consecutive days (oleation), followed on the evening of the fourth day by a hot bath and castor oil purgation (*virechana*). This is believed to remove lipid-soluble compounds as well as water-soluble toxins. Finally there is *shirodhara*, which involves lying down to receive a steady flow of medicated oil poured on the forehead to induce a deep state of relaxation.

Following is a description of one of the treatments used in the Maharishi Ayur-Ved *panchakarma* program:

> *Pizzicilli (Royal Treatment)*: Pizzicilli was designed for the royal families of ancient India to ensure a long life in perfect health. This luxurious treatment consists of an extensive full body massage by two technicians using a constant flow of warm herbalized oil. The oil penetrates deeply into the body tissues, softening and mobilizing impurities in preparation for *basti* treatment (an internal cleansing procedure).[12]

Chronotherapy

Ayurveda offers practical guidelines about how to create greater harmony among your *doshas* by changing your behavior patterns. Chronotherapy is the process of bringing your daily activity patterns into alignment with the natural metabolic rhythms and cycles your body goes through in each twenty-four-hour period. These natural patterns change somewhat with the seasons.

The general routine described on page 92 is recommended by Vivek Shanbhag, M.D. (Ayurveda), N.D., chairman of the department of Ayurvedic medicine at Bastyr University of Natural Health Sciences in Seattle.

SCIENTIFIC SUPPORT

Since Ayurveda is predominantly a person-specific approach, two individuals may have the exact same ailment and it could be attributed to different causes. They might be treated very differently, since what is curative for one person may be harmful to another with a different constitution. This makes it more challenging to design Western-style clinical trials for this tradition. Still, many studies have been conducted on specific Ayurvedic substances and on treatments for specific medical conditions.

A great deal of Ayurvedic research has been conducted in India in the last sixty to seventy years. This is a result of the influence of the British on the Indian educational system earlier this century and the teaching of Western scientific methods at Indian universities.

Today there are over forty research institutions in India that have conducted extensive clinical trials in Ayurvedic medicine, much of it supported by the government. However, most of this has been published in European and Indian scientific journals. In India, Ayurvedic research is published in both the mainstream medical journals and specific Ayurvedic journals, such as *Journal of Research in Ayurveda and Siddha*.

In the United States, proponents of Maharishi Ayur-Ved have provided most of the leadership in research. Much of their work has been with herbal products advocated by that group. This work has done a great deal to thrust Ayurveda into public awareness and is well documented in the book *Freedom from Disease* by Hari Sharma, M.D., professor of pathology and director, natural products research and cancer prevention, College of Medicine, Ohio State University.[13]

OAM-Funded Studies

The Office of Alternative Medicine at the National Institutes of Health has funded four studies in Ayurveda and related yoga practices.

Health Promotion. David Simon of the Sharp Institute for Human Potential and Mind/Body Medicine, San Diego, is comparing the effects of an Ayurvedic health promotion program with those of a conventional Western health promotion program for ninety enrollees in an HMO. Those in the Ayurveda program will follow a regimen of meditation, Ayurvedic diet, and hatha yoga postures. Those in the Western-style group will use progressive relaxation, a conventional Western diet with guidelines for low fat and salt, and aerobic exercise (brisk walking). A variety of physiological and behavioral outcomes will be compared for the two groups and for a third nonintervention group.

Parkinson's Disease. Bala V. Manyam of the Southern Illinois School of Medicine in Springfield, has been funded for a study of the effects of an Ayurvedic herbal formula on brain chemicals known to be affected in Parkinson's disease. This natural source of alkaloids that are believed effective against Parkinson's may be both cost-effective and beneficial for quality of life.

Heroin Addiction. Howard Shaffer of the North Charles Mental Health Research and Training Foundation in Cambridge, Massachusetts, is conducting a study of the use of hatha yoga in treatment of heroin addiction. The study will use hatha yoga in an outpatient methadone maintenance program and compare its effects to those of traditional group psychotherapy. Outcomes of interest include reducing alcohol and illicit drug use, reducing criminal activity, and increasing client retention in treatment.

Obsessive Compulsive Disorder. David Shannahoff-

> Khalsa of the Khalsa Foundation for Medical Sciences in Delmar, California, is studying the effects of a yogic breathing technique on obsessive compulsive disorder in adults and adolescents.

Laboratory Studies

Sharma and his colleagues have conducted basic research on two Ayurvedic herbal *rasayanas* that have historically been recommended for the treatment of cancer, gastrointestinal disorders, atherosclerosis, and other conditions. The substances in these studies are a version of a traditional metabolic tonic called *chyawanprash*—in this case, collectively called Maharishi Amrit Kalash (MAK-4 and MAK-5). They have shown several interesting physiological effects including powerful antioxidant (free radical scavenging) properties.

The ingredients in MAK-4 are raw sugar, ghee (clarified butter), Indian gallnut, Indian gooseberry, dried catkins, Indian pennywort, honey, nutgrass, white sandalwood, butterfly pea, shoeflower, aloewood, licorice, cardamom, cinnamon, cyperus, and turmeric. MAK-5 includes *Gymnema aurentiacum*, black musale, heart-leaved moonseed, *Sphaerantus indicus*, butterfly pea, licorice, *Vanda spatulatum*, elephant creeper, and Indian wild pepper.[14]

Findings of research with these formulas include reduction and elimination of tumors in mice,[15,16] reduced mortality in mice from a human cancer chemotherapy drug (Adriamycin),[17] increased lymphocyte proliferation (immune cell production) in animals,[18] and inhibition of the formation of cancer cells in human lung tumor cells.[19]

The finding about reducing the toxic effects of Adriamycin is very interesting in that it suggests that it may be possible to help humans tolerate more powerful doses of the drug. If this could be accomplished, cancer chemotherapy could possibly be made more effective, extending or even saving more lives.

Other findings include evidence that these substances are a thousand times more effective as antioxidants (free radical scavengers) than vitamins C and E and probucol (a cholesterol-lowering drug)[20]and significant reductions in platelet aggregation (clotting) in the blood of healthy people, which could prove useful in cardiovascular disorders.[21]

In 1987, researchers at MIT reported the effects of an herbal substance called Maharishi Ayur-Veda Maharasayana on experimentally induced colon cancer lesions in rats. Thirty to forty percent fewer lesions were found in rats given the herbal compound.[22]

Another herbal compound called Student Rasayana was found in animal studies to be a potent antioxidant that concentrates in the brain tissue. This may help explain apparent increases in intelligence that have been observed in children taking this compound.[23]

Sesame oil is commonly used in Ayurveda in daily self-massage, as a mouth rinse for oral hygiene, and in *panchakarma*. Anticancer properties have been found in sesame oil. One study showed inhibition of human colon cancer cell growth.[24] Another study found it suppressed the growth of cultured human malignant melanoma cells to a greater extent than did normal human melanocytes.[25]

Studies in Humans

A Multistrategy Program. Like other holistically oriented medical traditions, Ayurveda uses multiple forms of intervention to restore or promote health. One interesting study examined the effects of such a multistrategy program on chronic illnesses. The study included people with chronic headache, chronic constipation, chronic sinusitis, eczema, rheumatoid arthritis, hyperten-

Innovations in Surgery

The ancient textbook of Ayurvedic medicine, *Susruta Samhita*, named 1,120 diseases and described 127 different surgical instruments. Ancient Ayurvedic surgeons used many creative and exotic techniques. One method for suturing tissue together after surgery involved the use of tiger ants. The ants would be placed on the incision and would bite into the tissue on each side. Their two opposing fangs would work like a staple, binding the wound together. The surgeon would then cut off their heads, thus leaving the staple in place. Modern-day researchers have found that the ants release a secretion from their fangs that helps in wound healing.

sion, diabetes mellitus, bronchial asthma, chronic bronchitis, and psoriasis. A three-month program of treatments was provided to 126 adults in the Netherlands.[26]

The treatments included an individualized nutrition program, Maharishi Ayur-Ved herbal preparations, and behavioral guidelines for daily routines. The nutritional programs were tailored according to each person's individual constitution (*tridosha*) as well as their specific disease. In addition, the Maharishi Ayur-Ved herbal preparations were disease-specific, prepared according to traditional Ayurvedic formulas.

Other interventions included *panchakarma* (physiological purification therapy), *asanas* (yoga exercises used as neuromuscular integration therapy), and *marma* therapy (a form of pressure point massage therapy). Thirty patients used various of these therapies and 107 patients practiced the TM technique during the program.

Results indicated that 79 percent of patients experienced improvement, 14 percent showed no change, and 7 percent worsened. Each of the ten medical conditions being studied showed either highly significant improvement or strong trends toward improvement. The researchers reported complete cures for ten patients with the following conditions: rheumatoid arthritis, chronic bronchitis, eczema, chronic constipation, headache, and chronic sinusitis.

In a study such as this it is impossible, of course, to say how much each intervention contributed to the collective outcome. Also, the contribution of each form may have varied among individuals in the study. Studies like this are consistent, however, with the perspective that Ayurveda as a package of multiple strategies has benefit and there may be synergistic effects yet to be understood.

Panchakarma. In a study of the effects of *panchakarma* on risk factors for heart disease, thirty-one adults participated in a three- to five-day program. The treatment included oleation (use of clarified butter), *virechana* (purgation), *abhyanga* (medicated whole body massage), *shirodhara* (flow of medicated oil on the forehead), *swedna* (herbalized fomentation), *nasya* (nasal administration of herbs), and *basti* (herbalized enemas). Results three months after the treatment showed an 80-percent increase in VIP (a vasodilator), acute reduction in total cholesterol in all participants, reduction in lipid peroxide (a measure of free radical damage), and significant reduction in anxiety.[27]

In a controlled study of *panchakarma* involving 142 participants, those who underwent the program were found to report significant improvements in well-being, energy and vitality, strength and stamina, appetite and digestive patterns, and reduction of previous complaints as compared with controls. There were also significant reductions in anxiety, depression, and fatigue and an increase in vigor.[28]

Diabetes. A study examined the hypoglycemic and hypolipidemic effects of a Maharishi Ayur-Ved antidiabetic herbal formula (MA-471).[29] Forty-one patients with non-insulin-dependent diabetes participated. The patients fell into three groups: nine who were previously untreated and received the herbs only, twenty-three who had previously controlled their condition with oral hypoglycemic agents (OHA) and were switched to the herbs, and nine with previously uncontrolled symptoms while using OHA who added the herbs.

The official standards set by the American Diabetes Association (ADA) were used to evaluate the degree of patients' control over their condition. Within three months over 70 percent of the patients had achieved control rated as acceptable or good by the ADA standards. The greatest degree of improvement was found in the nineteen patients who had diabetes mellitus for less than five years. Benefits included reduction in other symptoms as well, such as weakness, appetite, polyuria, muscle pain, joint pain, constipation, palpitation, insomnia, and sense of well-being. The only side effect reported was a mild softening of stools.

Acne Vulgaris. A double-blind, placebo-controlled study was conducted for the effects of an Ayurvedic formula called *shankha bhasma*, a traditional Ayurvedic formula, in treating acne vulgaris. Two hundred eighty patients were assigned to groups based on their *prakriti*. Results of the four-week study showed that *vata* and *pitta* patients had significant improvement with the nontoxic treatment, while *kapha* patients did not. These results are explained by the fact that the formula has more action on *vata* and *pitta* metabolism.[30]

MAK-5 Studies. A double-blind, placebo-controlled study examined the effects of MAK-5 in forty-six people with hay fever. Conducted over four weeks at the peak of the hay fever season, the study found significant reductions in allergy symptoms in those taking this herbal *rasayana*.[31]

A study with nine people who took MAK-5 for three months found a significant decrease in Substance P (a neurotransmitter), suggesting that this herbal formula may relieve pain and help relieve pulmonary and gastrointestinal inflammation with no toxic effects.[32]

In a double-blind study of the effects of this *rasayana* on vision, forty-eight males over thirty-five were randomly assigned to receive MAK-5 or a placebo. All participants were practitioners of TM. After several weeks of treatment, those receiving the herbs showed significant improvement in a perceptual task involving the ability to locate symbols in a cluttered array. The researchers suggested that the herbs may also enhance the capacity for attention or alertness, thereby slowing or even reversing the effects of aging on cognitive functioning.[33]

Sesame Oil Mouth Rinse. The effects of using a daily sesame oil mouth rinse, a traditional Ayurvedic *rasayana*, was studied on a group of twenty-five healthy people. A significant decrease in growth of oral bacteria was found, suggesting this method may be an important approach to preventing periodontal disease, the major cause of tooth loss in adults.[34]

STRENGTHS AND LIMITATIONS

According to the historical texts, the primary aim of Ayurveda is prevention. It is first of all devoted to analysis of the healthy person and prescribing regimens to keep them healthy. The goal is to bring them to a higher and higher level of health, ultimately a state of perfect health, where they are fully creative, blissful, and actually enlightened.

Another strong interest is in extending the life span by activating and supporting the body's capacity for self-repair. The classical Ayurvedic teachings say that we have the potential to live much beyond what we consider to be a normal life span.

While cure of illness has theoretically been a secondary aim, Ayurveda is said by its proponents to do well with chronic, metabolic, and stress-related conditions. Because of scant clinical research, however, it is difficult to evaluate its effectiveness with many conditions.

A partial listing of conditions commonly treated by Ayurveda includes acid stomach, allergies, anxiety, asthma, arthritis, chronic fatigue syndrome, colds, colitis, constipation, depression, diabetes, flu, heart disease, hypertension, immune system disorders, inflammatory diseases, insomnia, irritable bowel syndrome, liver problems, menstrual cramps, neurological disorders, obesity, premenstrual syndrome, skin problems, and ulcers.

Limitations would include traumatic injuries, acute pain, diseases that are in an advanced stage, and those requiring surgery (although surgery is part of Ayurveda's history—see page 81). Generally, the earlier one is in a disease process, where there is less severe trauma to the integrity of the body, the more likely Ayurveda is to be successful.

Many practitioners argue that Ayurveda can help a great deal in reducing the side effects of toxic allopathic drug treatments (such as cancer chemotherapy) or speed recovery from surgery by rebalancing the body's *tridosha* and helping its self-repair mechanisms to function more efficiently.

THE PRACTITIONER-PATIENT RELATIONSHIP

Ayurveda does not rely on the practitioner as a treater or healer. Rather, he or she performs the initial diagnosis and then makes recommendations for dietary changes, herbal support, and perhaps other lifestyle changes. The bulk of the responsibility for treatment is on the patient through his or her daily living habits.

This is not to imply that the relationship is unimportant in Ayurveda, however. The original Ayurvedic teachings hold that the consciousness of the physician will have impact on that of the patient. Therefore it is imperative that the practitioner have the purest of intentions in order for the patient to get better. While the relationship is important from the point of view of reinforcing this clear intention as a foundation for healing, it is not considered the vehicle of treatment as such.

Typically the initial consultation is the longest, lasting from forty-five to ninety minutes. Often there are only one or two follow-up consultations, spaced several weeks or even months apart, to monitor progress. These will usually be briefer office visits.

Pitta-Pacifying But Not Vata-Aggravating Diet

Fruits
YES: Sweet fruits, avocado, coconut, figs, dark grapes, mango, sweet oranges, sweet pineapples, sweet plums, prunes
NO: Sour fruits, apricots, berries, bananas, cherries, cranberries, grapefruit, green grapes, lemons, sour oranges, papaya, peaches, sour pineapples, persimmon, sour plums (*Vata* aggravating: apples, melons, pears, pomegranate, dried fruits)

Vegetables
YES: Sweet and bitter vegetables, asparagus, cucumber, green beans, leafy greens*, lettuce*, okra, parsley*, sprouts*, zucchini
NO: Pungent vegetables, beets, carrots, eggplant, garlic, onions, peas, hot peppers, radishes, spinach, tomatoes (*Vata* aggravating: raw vegetables, broccoli, brussels sprouts, cabbage, cauliflower, celery, eggplant, mushrooms, peas, potatoes)

Grains
YES: Cooked oats, basmati rice, white rice, wheat
NO: Buckwheat, corn, millet, dry oats, brown rice, rye (*Vata* aggravating: barley)

Animal Products
YES: Chicken or turkey white meat, egg whites, shrimp (small amount), venison
NO: Beef, egg yolk, lamb, pork, seafood (*Vata* aggravating: rabbit)

Legumes
YES: Mung beans, tofu (*Vata* aggravating: all others)

Nuts/Seeds	NO nuts except coconut NO seeds except sunflower and pumpkin
Sweeteners	NO molasses, white sugar, or honey. All others okay.
Condiments	NO spices except coriander, cinnamon, cardamom, fennel, turmeric, and a little black pepper
Dairy	YES: Unsalted butter, cottage cheese, ghee, milk NO: Buttermilk, cheese, sour cream, yogurt
Oils	YES: Coconut, olive, sunflower, soy NO: Almond, corn, safflower, sesame
Other	2 tablespoons aloe vera juice 3 times a day

* in moderation with oil dressing

EVALUATING PERSONAL RESULTS

Evaluation of progress is based on both the patient's subjective reports of symptoms and the practitioner's assessment through the various forms of diagnosis. Most practitioners keep notes about each patient and record the impressions yielded by the diagnostic techniques for future comparison.

Some practitioners use laboratory blood, urine, and stool tests before and after treatment to help in evaluating results.

RELATIONSHIP TO OTHER FORMS OF MEDICINE

Generally Ayurveda is comfortably used as complementary or supportive to other forms of medicine. For example, as mentioned earlier, there is experimental evidence that some of its herbs may hold the potential to help cancer patients tolerate chemotherapy better, including reducing its toxic effects.

Since Ayurveda works by strengthening and balancing the body's healing mechanisms, it is not likely to conflict with other forms of medicine. One possible exception might be with other traditions that also use an herbal approach. It is probably not wise to mix herbal treatments from multiple traditions such as Chinese medicine, naturopathy, and Ayurveda. The practitioners who prescribe them may have specific metabolic processes in mind and may be working at cross purposes.

As with allopathy, you should discuss any medicines or herbs you are already taking with any practitioner of Ayurveda with whom you are working.

COSTS

The cost of consultations varies widely. An initial consultation may range from $40 to $100 or more, depending in part on the credentials and licensing of the practitioner. Follow-up visits will usually be proportionately less, depending on the time involved. Since there are usually few follow-up visits, Ayurveda tends to be relatively inexpensive in terms of professional services.

The cost of herbs may vary from $10 to $50 per month. Herbs can usually be purchased directly from the practitioner but are also available in health food stores and some oriental spice shops.

Specialized programs such as *panchakarma* can vary tremendously in cost, depending on the range of services and accommodations involved.

Insurance coverage will generally be limited to those licensed health care providers who are ordinarily covered because of their other qualifications and can incorporate Ayurveda into their regular office practice.

CHOOSING A PRACTITIONER

Ayurveda can be practiced by members of all health care disciplines as well as by health educators or consultants. The advantage to working with someone who is trained in another tradition, such as an M.D., naturopath, acupuncturist, or chiropractor, is of course the ability to integrate their expertise with those other areas. This might also help with insurance coverage. There is currently no national standard for certification of practitioners.

Extent of Training

There is a tremendous contrast between training in India and what is available in the West. In India the minimum standard for Ayurvedic physicians is a 5½-year degree, the Bachelor of Ayurvedic Medicine and Surgery (B.A.M.S.). There are close to two hundred such programs. Western-style medical schools also offer specializations in Ayurveda on a par with those in gynecology, neurology, cardiology, and so on. Indian M.D. degrees always list the specialty in parentheses, such as, in this case, "M.D. (Ayurveda)."

Western-trained practitioners generally have far less training, which raises the question of how much is needed for a person to be considered competent as a consultant or practitioner of this tradition. According to Deepak Chopra, M.D., "I think for somebody who is already a health professional seeing patients on an ongoing basis and has a theoretical framework that he is using to treat patients, it doesn't take that long to grasp the concepts. . . . General principles like prescribing *panchakarma*, body types, giving the appropriate diet, sensory modulation, aroma therapy, all these are pretty easy to grasp."

On the other hand, he adds, "One component of Ayurveda that takes a long time to fully grasp is the knowledge of Ayurvedic pharmacology and herbs. That only comes through experience. You can't memorize the properties of herbs and do it that way. Pulse diagnosis also takes a long time."[35]

Dr. Shanbhag concurs, offering the opinion that Ayurveda is very much a subjective science and that the experience of the practitioner is key. "If they have had less than three years of clinical experience, I would consider them a novice. That's my personal feeling. . . . The more time they have spent in it, the more contact with patients, and the more Ayurvedic logic they have used, they can train themselves." He suggests that a practitioner needs to have seen a minimum of a thousand people under close supervision to become skilled at pulse and *prakriti* diagnosis.[36]

Training Programs

Most of the programs listed below are also associated with clinics that offer individual consultation, sell Ayurvedic products, and conduct *panchakarma* detoxification programs.

The Ayurvedic Institute in Albuquerque was founded by Dr. Vasant Lad, formerly a professor of internal medicine and medical director of an Ayurvedic hospital in India. The institute offers training programs to professionals and laypersons. Programs include an eight-month course with clinical supervision, opportunities for correspondence study, and weekend seminars. Address: P.O. Box 23445, Albuquerque, NM 87192–1445, phone (505) 291–9698, FAX (505) 294–7572.

The American Institute of Vedic Studies, founded by David Frawley, O.M.D., offers a program of study for health care professionals in alliance with Ayurvedic schools in India. The training consists of a correspondence course, followed by a two-week intensive held in Santa Fe focusing on Ayurvedic massage and *panchakarma* therapy. The program can be applied toward continuing education credits for chiropractic physicians. Address: P.O. Box 8357, Santa Fe, NM 87504–8357, phone (505) 983–9385.

College of Maharishi Ayur-Ved, Maharishi International University offers a training program limited to licensed primary health care providers (mainly doctors of medicine, chiropractic, naturopathy, and osteopathy). The training involves two fifty-hour courses taken in residence at the college, each given over a one-week period. Other trainings are offered in other parts of the country. At this writing about three hundred practitioners have been certified. Address: 1000 4th St., DB-1155 Fairfield, IA 52557–1155, phone (515) 472–7000, FAX (375) 472–1189.

Bastyr University of Natural Health Sciences offers a specialization in Ayurvedic medicine within its four-year doctoral program for naturopathic physicians. The degree is designated "N.D. (Ayurveda)." Naturopaths are licensed as primary care providers in many states (see Chapter 4). Address: 144 N.E. 54th St., Seattle, WA 98105, phone (206) 523–9585, FAX (206) 527–4763.

The Center for Mind/Body Medicine has both residential and outpatient programs. Developed under the guidance of Deepak Chopra, M.D., it also provides education and training programs in Ayurveda for laypeople and health care providers. Address: P.O. Box 1048, La Jolla, CA 92038, phone (619) 794–2425, FAX (619) 794–2440.

The American School of Ayurvedic Sciences is headed by Virender Sodhi, M.D. (India), N.D., a former medical school professor in India and a former faculty member at Bastyr Univer-

Early to Bed, Early to Rise . . .

Dr. Vivek Shanbhag of the Department of Ayurvedic Medicine, Bastyr University, Seattle, recommends the following daily routine to stay in harmony with the cycles of the body:

Morning

1. Arise early, preferably 30 minutes before sunrise.
2. Evacuate bowels and bladder.
3. Clean and brush teeth.
4. Clean and scrape the tongue with a tongue scraper or toothbrush.
5. Clean the eyes by sprinkling with cold water.
6. Drink a glass of clean water at room temperature with a teaspoon of raw, uncooked honey or drink a glass of fruit juice at room temperature.
7. Warm sesame oil massage to head, body, and soles of feet 7 to 10 minutes (at least twice a week, especially during the weekend).
8. Brief warm-up exercises, stretches, yoga postures, or 5 to 10 Sun Salutes for 10 to 12 minutes.
9. Bath or shower preferably with a minimum of warm water. Begin with a comfortable temperature and gradually lower the temperature as low as possible. Never wash your head with warm water.
10. Wear clean and comfortable clothes suitable to the season and activity.
11. Breathing exercises or *pranayama*.
12. Concentration and relaxation exercises or meditation.
13. Breakfast consisting of diet balanced according to your individual psychosomatic constitution, daily requirement, and season.
14. Work or study.

Midmorning

Drink of water or herb tea and snack of fruit or fig bar.

Afternoon

1. Lunch consisting of diet balanced according to your individual psychosomatic constitution, daily requirement, and season.
2. Brief rest after lunch for about 10 to 15 minutes.
3. Work or study.

Midafternoon

Drink of water or herb tea and snack of fruit or fig bar.

Evening

1. Physical exercise for 20 to 30 minutes. Preferable exercises are Sun Salutations, yoga postures, swimming, or fast walking.
2. Leave an interval of 20 to 30 minutes in between exercise and dinner.
3. Dinner consisting of diet balanced according to psychosomatic constitution, daily requirement, and season.
4. Brief walk for 15 to 20 minutes.
5. Relaxing and recreational activity.
6. Early to bed (leave about a 60- to 90-minute gap in between dinner and going to bed).

sity of Natural Health Sciences, Seattle. The institute offers several levels of training, including extended training programs for primary health care providers as well as specialized courses in Ayurvedic nutrition, yoga, and massage. Address: 10025 N.E. 4th, Bellevue, WA 98004, phone (206) 453–8022, FAX (206) 451–2670.

YogAyu is directed by Vivek Shanbhag, M.D. (Ayurveda), N.D., who is also chairman of the department of Ayurvedic medicine at Bastyr University of Natural Health Sciences, Seattle. The center offers a two-week summer intensive training program in Ayurvedic therapies. Address: 23700 Edmonds Way, Edmonds, WA 98026, phone (206) 542–3528.

The Ayurveda Holistic Center of New York, directed by Swami Sada Shiva Tirtha, offers a correspondence course, a thirty-six-hour training course, and a supervised internship in Ayurveda. Address: 82A Bayville Ave., Bayville, NY 11709, phone/FAX (516) 628–8200.

Vedic Sciences Institute, directed by Deva Treadway, Ph.D., offers a forty-five-hour course with a hundred-hour supervised internship leading to the designation "Certified Ayurvedist (C.Av.)." Treadway studied in India and has developed an approach called American Ayurveda. Address: P.O. Box 2537, Jupiter, FL 33468–2537, phone (407) 745–2164.

Other Organizations

Maharishi Ayur-Ved Medical Association publishes a newsletter for physicians, including information about physician training programs. Address: RR4 Box 503, Fairfield, IA 52556, phone (515) 472–9580, FAX (515) 472–2496.

Maharishi Ayur-Ved Products International publishes a catalog called *Total Health*, provides information, and sells herbal Ayurveda products. Address: P.O. Box 49667, Colorado Springs, CO 80949, phone (800) 255–8332, FAX (719) 260–7400.

Conclusion

With no standardized way of credentialing practitioners of Ayurveda, there is a very wide range of expertise. The best way to determine the preparation of a practitioner is to inquire about the extent of their training and experience and what certifications or degrees they may have from training programs that support this tradition. Of course, the recommendations of others, as well as years of experience, may help in making this assessment.

One criterion suggested by Dr. Cravatta is the practitioner's own appearance: If they look healthy and vital themselves, they are more likely to understand the principles well. Since Ayurveda is noninvasive and nontoxic, it is essentially a risk-free approach you can explore to determine whether it is right for you.

CHAPTER 4

NATUROPATHIC MEDICINE: THE GREAT CORNUCOPIA

"There is really but one healing force in existence and that is Nature herself, which means the inherent restorative power of the organism to overcome disease."

—BENEDICT LUST

Naturopathic medicine traces its roots back thousands of years to many ancient cultures. In a sense, this is the oldest medicine known to man, since most medicine before this century was based essentially on natural substances and natural processes.

The origins of naturopathy in the United States are attributed to Benedict Lust, who came to this country in 1896 from Germany to practice and teach the hydrotherapy methods made popular by an Austrian priest named Sebastian Kneipp. Lust had cured himself of tuberculosis using Kneipp's therapy of hot and cold water treatments and was an enthusiastic advocate of natural therapies.

After completing his own medical training, Lust founded the first school of naturopathic medicine in New York City, which graduated its first class in 1902. The training was expanded to include botanical medicine, nutritional therapy, physiotherapy, psychology, homeopathy, and manual manipulation therapies. During this same period, Dr. James Foster founded a similar school in Idaho, spawning acceptance of this profession in the Northwest. Together, Lust and Foster named their profession naturopathy. Other labels that have been used for this tradition are nature cure and natural medicine.

The young profession grew rapidly and naturopathic medical conventions in the 1920s were attended by as many as ten thousand practitioners. There were over twenty naturopathic colleges and the profession was licensed in most states. However, in the 1940s and 50s it began to decline, overshadowed by the tremendous growth in allopathic medicine, the burgeoning pharmaceutical industry, and the rise in prominence of the American Medical Association.

Naturopathy virtually disappeared until a resurgence of popular interest in holistic and natural methods of healing in the 1970s and 80s. It has undergone a rebirth and in today's climate of unprecedented interest in natural healing and disaffection with conventional medicine, it once again is on the ascent. Currently, just under a thousand naturopaths practice in the United States.

Education

In 1987 the Council on Naturopathic Medical Education was recognized by the federal government as the accrediting body for naturopathic medical colleges, of which there are currently four: Bastyr University of Natural Health Sciences, Seattle, Washington; National College of Naturopathic Medicine, Portland, Oregon; Southwest College of Naturopathic Medicine and Health Sciences, Scottsdale, Arizona; and The Canadian College of Naturopathic Medicine, Toronto, Ontario, Canada.

Modern naturopathic physicians undergo a four-year education and are trained as primary health care providers with preparation in preventive medicine and natural therapeutics, as well as diagnosing, managing, and treating early onset chronic degenerative disease.

The medical education of naturopaths is comparable to that of allopathic (conventional) medical schools in terms of basic training in the biomedical sciences. This includes anatomy, physiology, biochemistry, pathology, microbiology, immunology, pharmacology, clinical and physical diagnosis, laboratory diagnosis, cardiology, neurology, radiology, minor surgery, obstetrics, gynecology, pediatrics, and dermatology.[1] The points at which naturopathy and allopathy diverge are in the underlying philosophy of health and illness and in the types of treatments that are taught once the foundation in basic medical sciences is established.

KEY PRINCIPLES

Lust's early writings include a description of basic principles of naturopathy that could be considered remarkably contemporary. He describes the "principles, aim, and program of the nature cure" as follows:

> The natural system for curing disease is based on a return to nature in regulating the diet, breathing, exercising, bathing and the employment of various forces to eliminate the poisonous products in the system, and so raise the vitality of the patient to a proper standard of health.[2]

Lust's program included three major components: (1) elimination of evil habits (overeating, alcoholic drinks, drugs, use of tea, coffee, meat eating, improper hours of living, sexual and social aberrations, and so on); (2) corrective habits (correct breathing, exercise, right mental attitude, and other things in moderation); and (3) new principles of living (proper fasting, selection of food, hydrotherapy, light and air baths, mud baths, osteopathy, chiropractic and other forms of manipulation, mineral salts, steam baths, and so on).

With regard to the healing force of nature, Lust posed the question, "Can this power be appropriated and guided more readily by extrinsic or intrinsic methods? That is to say, is it more amenable to combat disease by irritating drugs, vaccines and serums employed by superstitious moderns, or by the bland intrinsic congenial forces of Natural therapeutics, that are employed by this new school of medicine, that is Naturopathy, which is the only orthodox school of medicine? Are not these natural forces much more orthodox than the artificial resources of the druggist? The practical application of these natural agencies, duly suited to individual case, are true signs that the art of healing has been elaborated by the aid of absolutely harmless, congenial treatments."

Lust's view of naturopathy as the only "orthodox" form of medicine helps illustrate just how subjective such terms as "orthodox," "mainstream," and "alternative" are today.

A Unifying Philosophy

From the time of Lust onward, naturopaths may be described as eclectic, meaning that they combine natural interventions from a variety of medical traditions. According to Michael Murray, N.D., of Bastyr University of Natural Health Sciences in Seattle, a well-known lecturer and writer on natural health, "I look at the naturopathic medicine of today as being an amalgamation of all the healing arts of the past, but with the modern scientific validation. It's a kind of blending of old world thinking with new world thinking."[3]

This eclecticism has led to some confusion about what distinguishes naturopathy from other traditions. In the 1980s an effort was undertaken by the American Association of Naturopathic Physicians (AANP) to clarify the unique frame of reference of naturopathic medicine and define it in terms of a unifying philosophy rather than simply the modalities it uses.

Jared Zeff, N.D., L.Ac., academic dean at National College of Naturopathic Medicine in Portland, Oregon, was one of those who drafted the statement for the AANP. He states: "What we really do isn't just collect arcane therapies. We practice medicine from a philosophy that is really quite ancient." The philosophy, which was articulated by Hippocrates, is that the body heals itself and the task of the physician is to support this inherent healing potential.[4]

The unifying philosophy of naturopathy is contained in the following six principles:

Vis Medicatrix Naturae **(The Healing Power of Nature).** The healing process is ordered and intelligent. The body has the inherent ability—the vitality—not only to heal itself and restore health, but also to ward off disease. Illness is not caused simply by an invasion of external agents or germs, but is a manifestation of the organism's attempt to defend and heal itself. The physician's role is to identify and remove agents blocking the healing process, bolster the patient's healing capacity, and support the creation of a healthy internal and external environment.

Treat the Whole Person. A person's health status results from a complex interaction of physical, mental, emotional, genetic, spiritual, environmental, social, and other factors. The harmonious functioning of all these aspects is essential to health. Within the body, the different systems are intimately connected, dynamically balanced. *Dis-ease* or imbalance in one part directly affects all other parts of the whole. There is never a single cause for disease. All the pieces must be integrated in order to create a whole picture of an individual and his or her illness. Therapy can then be directed at underlying as well as immediate causative factors, thus treating the whole person.

Primum No Nocere **(First Do No Harm).** In respecting the inherent ability of the organism to heal itself, the physician must be ever mindful of the consequences or side effects of treatment.

Kathleen

Kathleen, thirty-five, had been diagnosed with membranous cystitis, a bladder inflammation commonly thought to be incurable. She was given a cleansing and detoxifying diet, did hydrotherapy treatments, took a homeopathic remedy, and was given herbs for cleaning and healing the bladder. After three weeks the bladder problem had disappeared.

The more gentle and noninvasive the therapy, the less disruptive it will be to the patient. Whenever possible, suppression of symptoms is avoided, as this may interfere with the healing process.

Tolle Causam (**Identify and Treat the Cause**). Illness does not occur without cause and symptoms (nausea, rash, headache) are not the cause. Symptoms are signals that the body is out of balance. They are an expression of the body's attempt to heal itself. Causes originate on many levels, but are more often found in the patient's lifestyle, diet, habits, or emotional state. When only the symptoms are treated, the underlying causes remain and the patient may develop a more serious, chronic condition.

Prevention Is the Best Cure. Health is a reflection of how we choose to live. Physicians help patients recognize their choices and how those choices affect their health. The doctor assesses risk factors and hereditary susceptibility to disease and makes appropriate intervention to prevent illness. One cannot be healthy in an unhealthy environment and it is the responsibility of both the physician and patient to create a world in which humanity may thrive.

Docere (**Doctor as Teacher**). The original meaning of the word *doctor* was "teacher." One of a physician's responsibilities is to educate the patient and encourage self-responsibility. The physician must recognize each patient as an individual responding to and shaping his or her own environment. A cooperative doctor-patient relationship has inherent therapeutic value.

Healing and Symptoms

In the naturopathic perspective, healing is not a matter of waging war against disease by introducing extraordinary outside resources to attack the pathogens. Rather, it is a matter of supporting the body's own inherent healing mechanisms to help them actualize their highest potential.

An interesting illustration of naturopathic thought is seen in its perspective on one of our most common symptoms, inflammation. According to Zeff, the inflammatory response is one of the body's healing mechanisms and should not be routinely suppressed.

"If you look at what inflammation is," he states, "what you'll see is it's primarily based upon increased blood flow and activation of the immune system. The body *made* the inflammation to *heal* itself. If that response is sufficient to carry away the disturbance, and usually it is if it's an acute situation, then the inflammation is followed by a discharge, resolution, and return to normalization.

"But if the disturbance continues, the inflammation becomes chronic and ultimately degenerative, and that's when you might see ulceration or even tumor formation. From that observation comes a kind of logical understanding of how to intervene, when and what tools to use—based upon the philosophy of *working with* the body's self-healing potential."

An example of the naturopathic view speaks to the most common ailment known to man: the cold, a simple viral infection. Most of us have developed the attitude that there is nothing we can really do about a cold other than try and live with the symptoms. What this entails is taking remedies to suppress or eliminate them, such as a decongestant for the nasal congestion.

We want to be rid of the swelling and congestion and runny nose, as if to say, "Okay, so I have this cold. But that doesn't mean I have to suffer with these horrible, messy symptoms. I'll take this decongestant and the cold will eventually pass." So we take a substance designed to suppress that particular symptom.

If we understand, however, that the symptoms themselves *are the very mechanisms the body uses to fight the viral infection*, then we would not want to interfere with them, but would want to give them all the support we can to enhance and strengthen their activity.

During a cold, our immune cells are activated to fight off a virus. Histamine is released by mast cells in order to cause swelling and inflammation *so that greater blood circulation is possible, bringing more white cells in to fight the viruses*. The body creates an abundance of mucus, which helps to flush out the membranes and discharge the waste products of this healing process.

Certainly it is more pleasant in the short run to be able to take a drug to suppress our symptoms, and this may even enable us to go back to work sooner or partake more fully of other things we value. It represents a kind of conquest of the body. But, naturopathy asks, at what cost? And what does our conquest of symptoms reveal to us about our relationship to our bodies and where they stand among our priorities?

In the naturopathic perspective, the body is working hard to follow its own inborn healing strategy, which includes the production of histamine. Hence, when we take a decongestant or an antihistamine, we are directly combating the body's best efforts to heal. And the ominous fact is that the body learns. Immune responses become conditioned over time. Repeated experiences of having a certain healing response suppressed may lead to the eventual weakening and elimination of that ability. Yet, this is precisely what we do when we seek to suppress symptoms.

Naturopaths do not enjoy flowing mucus and their approach

is not to just resign and let nature take its course. Rather, the effort is to usher nature along more expeditiously. This will of course speed the recovery process and the elimination of symptoms more quickly.

There are several natural means to support these efforts. For example, we might:

(1) drink more liquid to aid the flushing out of the membranes
(2) take vitamin C and zinc to enhance the functioning of the white cells in pursuing the viruses
(3) mix what the natural health advocate and author Dana Ullman calls a "lemon cocktail" consisting of fresh squeezed lemon juice (for its vitamin C content) with warm water and a pinch of cayenne pepper to help stimulate mucous membranes, loosen mucus, and increase circulation
(4) mix an herb tea with herbs known to help the body fight cold viruses, such as rose hips, hyssop, ginger, pepper, mint, and sage
(5) breathe vapors from eucalyptus, a powerful antiseptic and expectorant, by placing a few drops of oil in a bowl of hot water, putting a towel over your head to trap the vapors, and inhaling them
(6) eat garlic for its antiviral and immune-stimulating properties
(7) take a homeopathic dose of onions, called *allium cepa*, to provoke and accelerate the body's efforts to bring the drainage to a conclusion[5]

Certainly there are cases, especially in advanced stages of disease, where the body's symptom strategies break down and are unable to overcome a disease process. This of course is where the heroic measures of high-tech and modern pharmaceutical medicine can save lives or at least help maintain a better quality of life. Naturopaths readily acknowledge these strengths of allopathic medicine and usually have positive collaborative relationships with other physicians.

Sharon

Sharon, twenty-five, had been experiencing acute abdominal pain. She was taken to an emergency room by her boyfriend and was subsequently diagnosed with gallstones and cholecystitis, inflammation of the gallbladder. She was scheduled for surgery to have her gallbladder removed.

Sharon sought a consultation with a naturopath to see if she could avoid the surgery. He palpated her gallbladder and found it to be extremely tender, consistent with the diagnosis she had received. He immediately gave her a homeopathic remedy and an acupuncture treatment. He put her on a zero fat diet and instructed her in daily use of hydrotherapy on her abdomen. By the time she left the office an hour later, 90 percent of the pain was gone.

Over the next several days as she followed the recommendations her discomfort diminished further. Within four days she had returned to work and after a week she had no more pain. With the help of some herbs intended to improve stomach function, her digestion began to improve and she continued this regime for six weeks with no further symptoms.

She was also given herbs to help clean the liver and was told that over time proper metabolism will dissolve the stones. The total cost of treatment was about $200. The cost of the surgery was estimated at $25,000.

Detoxification

One of the most important processes in promoting or optimizing overall health is detoxification. This is what Lust meant when he said "eliminate the poisonous products in the system, and so raise the vitality of the patient."[6] Modern-day researchers know that toxins accumulating in the internal organs and the blood can impair organ function as well as immune function. They are at the root of modern maladies such as environmental illness and play a role in many chronic illnesses.

Toxemia, the buildup in the body of toxic substances, can also be generated internally by a buildup of waste products that result from poor digestion. This is the common condition at the root of many of today's most common maladies.

Most digestive disturbances are caused by food intolerances and chronic stress. Both these factors result in poorer digestion (the stress response decreases blood flow to the gut and sends it to the brain and muscles for fight or flight). Thus the two most important steps to take to decrease toxic load in the body are to improve the diet (not supplementation, but food choice) and reduce stress.

Perspective on Modern Illnesses

Why do we have such an abundance of chronic and degenerative illnesses? To the naturopath, they result from an interaction of environmental changes, lifestyle choices, and the chronic overuse of certain forms of medicine. During the past 150 years we have introduced countless unnatural irritants into the environment and increasing health problems should be expected as a logical result. Yet, according to Zeff, most of modern medicine is based upon suppressing the inflammatory response. This practice has real implications for the health of the population at large.

"It's logical to the naturopathic mind that when you suppress the inflammatory response of an entire population you'll see increased degenerative and chronic disease," he observes. "So what we're seeing now, after the era in which the miracle antibiotics were introduced, is a vastly increased degree of chronic and degenerative disease, even in children."

There is no doubt that antibiotics have saved countless lives and this is not meant as a blanket condemnation of antibiotics. In fact, naturopaths have recently been granted authority to prescribe them in the state of Washington. What is of concern to the naturopath is that these and other modern drugs, if used indiscriminately, may have a cumulative weakening effect on the body's own healing mechanisms, which are not allowed to fully express themselves. Indeed, a 1982 report in the *American Journal of Medicine* found that antibiotics depress at least four components of the immune system.[7]

VARIETIES OF NATUROPATHIC PRACTICE

While all practitioners share the common philosophy and principles described earlier, there are shades of a spectrum of naturopathic practice. At one end of the spectrum are the approaches that could be considered purely vitalistic, and at the other end would be those that are biochemically oriented.

The Vitalistic Approach

The vitalistic school of thought is most closely aligned with the historic roots of naturopathy in terms of its emphasis on the body's natural healing power (*vis medicatrix naturae*). The body, with its inherent wisdom, directs any therapeutic process and therapies are given with the intention of evoking or working with these inherent healing abilities.

Thus at the core of the vitalistic orientation are the use of dietary change, hydrotherapy designed to improve blood flow to the digestive system, and stress reduction. All of these result in improved digestion, which is seen as a key in detoxifying the body and is necessary for the body's inherent healing abilities

Maureen

Maureen is a twenty-two-year-old student who had been suffering from constipation for nine months since returning from a trip to Mexico. Her bowel movements had been just once per week.

She was also three months pregnant. Her gastroenterologist had prescribed some stool softeners, which were not helping. He told her the next step was a colorectal examination but that there was a risk of miscarriage with the procedure.

David Field, N.D., L.Ac., describes his approach: "After taking a detailed case history, I gave her a flaxseed hull preparation as a fiber and instructed her to drink a quart of water in the morning and a quart in the afternoon.

"Suspecting an intestinal parasite, I gave her a probiotic formula with eight beneficial bacteria in it. She also took some fructo-oligosaccharides, which are a nutrient that the beneficial bacteria thrive on in the intestine. This protocol is to overwhelm the pathogens in the intestine with beneficial bacteria."

Maureen returned three weeks later reporting daily stools. The cost of treatment was $110 for the office visits and $40 per month for the supplements, which she will continue through at least the first six months of the pregnancy.

to be able to fully express themselves. The vital force is seen as the preeminent factor in healing and this approach, if followed thoroughly, generally brings a rapid improvement in most any chronic condition.

It is only after this level of intervention that the vitalistically oriented naturopath considers the use of herbs or other modalities for targeting specific symptoms. These are thought of as secondary or tertiary therapies to restore function that has been weakened or damaged. Indeed, in the history of naturopathy diet and hydrotherapy were originally taught as the basis of healing and herbs were added later.

The Biochemical Approach

Whereas the vitalistic approach focuses on general stimulation of the body as the first line of treatment, the more biochemically oriented naturopaths may more readily and liberally employ herbs and nutritional substances as the first line of treatment. Substances may be chosen on the basis of their biochemistry and their effects on specific symptoms or disease states.

This approach views naturopathy as an alternative to conventional medicine by virtue of its using substances that are more "biologically correct." However, consistent with allopathic thinking, it may still be both substance-oriented and symptom- or disease-oriented. It uses natural substances as "more gentle drugs."

In practice this approach tends to be more predominant than the vitalistic approach, as such biochemical thinking is a strong force in Western culture. While we may prefer natural rather than pharmaceutically manufactured substances, we still want to pop a pill for a symptom. The biochemical approach to naturopathy does lend itself well, however, to Western-style scientific research studies, so this is the direction much research is taking as the tradition seeks scientific validation.

Treatment Modalities

Below are descriptions of the major treatment modalities used in naturopathy. While all practitioners share the common philosophy and principles described earlier, any one of the following forms of intervention can become an area of specialization. Practitioners may also choose to specialize in a particular problem area such as pediatrics, allergies, or arthritis. Although naturopaths are trained as primary health care providers, the licensing laws of some states limit what modalities can be used.

Clinical Nutrition. This is the foundation of naturopathic medical practice. It includes dietary recommendations and nutritional supplementation with herbs, vitamins, minerals, and other substances. It may also include laboratory testing of bodily fluids to assess the nutritional status of the body and monitor change. Foods are considered not only for basic nourishment, but as potentially medicinal substances.

Physical Medicine. This involves the therapeutic manipulation of muscles, bones, and the spine. Other modalities include massage therapy, deep tissue bodywork, ultrasound, diathermy, exercise, and therapeutic use of electrical stimulation.

Hydrotherapy, which is one of the most celebrated of all naturopathic therapies, involves hot and cold moisture to the body to improve circulation. One common method is to use towels that are wrung out in hot and cold water and alternately applied to the body. The intense fluctuations in temperature serve to improve circulation to the stomach, liver, kidneys, and intestines, thereby improving digestion and elimination of metabolic waste. The toxic load on all the vital organs is reduced and the immune system is stimulated. This treatment is used with everything from ear infections to cancer.

Homeopathy. Homeopathic remedies are natural substances used to strengthen the body's vital force (life force, life energy), thereby helping the body to use its own resources to eliminate symptoms and illness. This is one of the more common specializations among naturopathic physicians.

Botanical Medicine. This involves the medicinal use of plant substances, also known as herbal medicine. Because these sub-

110

stances are organic, in their natural state rather than being chemically derived, they are more easily assimilated and integrated into the body's own chemistry, resulting in fewer side effects than pharmaceutically manufactured substances.

Naturopathic Obstetrics. This includes non-hospital-based, natural childbirth care and prenatal and postnatal care using modern diagnostic techniques. The emphasis is on using natural, noninvasive interventions in order to prevent complications.

Chinese Medicine. Many naturopaths are fully trained and licensed or certified in Chinese medicine, including herbs and acupuncture. This is another common specialization in naturopathic medical schools.

Ayurveda. Ayurveda is the world's oldest system of natural medicine. Its influence is growing in the West and it is an attractive specialty for many naturopaths. Bastyr University of Natural Health Sciences in Seattle has inaugurated a specialization in Ayurveda within its doctoral program, leading to the degree N.D. (Ayurveda).

Psychological Medicine. Counseling, psychotherapy, hypnotherapy, and behavioral medicine are often used to help patients deal with the psychological dimensions of health. Another important component of naturopathy is patient education for compliance with health-promoting lifestyle changes.

Environmental Medicine. Some naturopaths specialize in detoxification and immune restoration therapies for helping people overcome the burdens of toxic chemical exposure and buildup, which are a cause of many modern illnesses.

Minor Surgery. Naturopaths are trained to do minor in-office surgery (repair of superficial wounds, removal of foreign bodies, cysts, and other superficial masses) with local anesthesia.

Sandra

Sandra, a thirty-year-old business administrator with insulin-dependent diabetes, sought help for a large diabetic ulcer on her leg. In addition to being a blood sugar–related disease, diabetes is a vascular disease that involves the deterioration of small blood vessels. The extremities (legs and feet, arms and hands) often have problems of poor circulation and such ulcers are a common occurrence.

The practitioner gave her zinc, beta carotene, and a topical goldenseal cream to apply to the ulcer. He also recommended the use of hydrotherapy each night before bed to aid in the circulation problem. This involves first soaking the feet in warm water, then putting on a pair of cold wet socks, covered by a pair of dry wool socks, and going straight to bed.

After she followed this regime for three weeks the ulcer on Sandra's leg had disappeared. She continues the hydrotherapy treatment four times a week on a preventive basis.

As David Field, N.D., L.Ac., explains, the cold moisture has the effect of provoking the body's protective response of increasing peripheral circulation, especially in the feet and legs. Usually they become so warm during the night that the socks dry out and the person has to remove both pairs. The method is used commonly in diabetes and other problems associated with poor circulation in the extremities, including the hands.

There are no modalities that are exclusive or unique to naturopathic medicine as such. However, while many of these modalities are shared by other traditions, naturopaths hold that what distinguishes their practice is that it is guided by adherence to the six principles outlined earlier.

PROCEDURES AND TECHNIQUES

Many naturopaths use a previsit questionnaire, often mailed to the patient at the time the appointment is made. Then in the initial meeting the practitioner will use this as an aid in discussing complaints.

Typically the initial meeting takes about an hour and involves a thorough medical history and interview intended to evaluate all aspects of the person's lifestyle. This provides an important context for diagnosing and understanding the presenting problems. Standard diagnostic procedures including a physical exam and blood and urine tests may also be called for.

Some naturopaths use tests that are not used in conventional medicine, such as the urine indican test to determine the degree of intestinal putrefaction (undigested and decaying food) or toxemia, or the Heidelberg test, which measures stomach acidity, an indicator of digestive function.

What happens beyond the initial interview depends on the specialization of the practitioner. From here the process may move into a more detailed nutritional assessment if a clinical nutrition approach is being used. Or, in cases where the practitioner uses Chinese medicine, homeopathy, Ayurveda, or another approach, the next steps will follow accordingly. In general, follow-up meetings average about a half hour.

Most naturopaths practice office-based medicine. By philosophy, they use the least invasive therapy possible and rely heavily on patient education and lifestyle modification. Hence a substantial amount of time in appointments may be devoted to lifestyle assessment and counseling for changing to more health-promoting behaviors. Most view the professional relationship as involving teaching to some degree, since patient compliance with lifestyle recommendations (e.g., diet, exercise, relaxation) is often necessary for lasting improvement.

Although naturopaths have prescription rights for some classes of drugs in some states, in general they are not allowed to prescribe drugs. A notable exception is the state of Washington where they are allowed to prescribe antibiotics, thyroid medicines, progesterone, and some other drugs.

An excellent resource for the layperson for naturopathic approaches, including the use of herbs, vitamins, minerals, diet, and nutritional supplementation with over seventy common health problems, is *The Encyclopedia of Natural Medicine*, by Michael Murray, N.D., and Joseph Pizzorno, N.D. (Rocklin, CA: Prima Publishing, 1991, $18.95, available in bookstores).

SCIENTIFIC SUPPORT

This tradition bases its practice on both clinical experience and scientific research. Since it uses methods from a variety of traditions, the scientific support is often derived from other contexts—including mainstream academic institutions.

According to Dr. Murray, "A lot of the historical therapies and practices of naturopathic medicine are being validated by modern scientific inquiry. For example, naturopaths have been using vitamin E for its antioxidant and protective effects against heart disease for well over thirty years."

He adds, "One of the great myths that's promoted by the medical establishment is that natural medicine is not based upon science. . . . Most Americans are unaware of the tremendous body of scientific knowledge that supports the use of natural measures. In fact, when you look at the totality of evidence, there's a greater scientific rationale for the use of nutrition, herbal medicine, and other natural therapies for most common illnesses than there is for standard drug or surgical procedures."[8]

Indeed, a 1979 article published in the *Journal of the American Medical Association* concluded that in 90 percent of condi-

OAM-Funded Studies

Naturopathic principles are under scrutiny in two studies being funded by the Office of Alternative Medicine, National Institutes of Health.

Antioxidant Vitamins and Cancer. Kedarn Prasad of the University of Colorado Health Sciences Center, Denver, has been funded for a study of whether high doses of multiple antioxidant vitamins can improve the effectiveness of chemotherapy and radiation therapy in cancer. The hypothesis is that high doses of these natural substances may enhance the effects of the conventional forms of treatment on tumor cells and may also protect normal cells against adverse effects. (This study may also help explain why certain Ayurvedic and Chinese herbal substances have shown similar benefits in other research—see Chapters 2 and 3.)

Macrobiotic Diet and Cancer. Lawrence Kushi of the University of Minnesota School of Public Health is developing a collaborative study with the Kushi Foundation, one of the world's foremost centers for macrobiotic education. The study is designed to develop data collection procedures that can be used in formal clinical trials that will measure the impact of the macrobiotic diet on the course of cancer.

In addition, Bastyr University in Seattle has been named as a National Institutes of Health Exploratory Center for Alternative Medicine Research. Bastyr's Center for Alternative Treatments for HIV/AIDS has been funded to describe the forms and patterns of alternative therapy use by HIV/AIDS patients, to screen and evaluate those therapies, to provide training to alternative medical practitioners to evaluate therapies scientifically, and to educate the scientific biomedical community on alternative medical treatment of these patients.

Vincent

Vincent was a forty-five-year-old businessman suffering from chronic fatigue syndrome for three and a half years. He described himself as modestly successful and not a workaholic. He had little mental alertness, was able to work only ten hours a week, and was in bed the rest of the time. He had taken three years of vitamin therapy and had been taking allergy shots for twenty years. He brought twenty-five pages of lab work with him to the naturopath's office.

A hypoallergenic diet was prescribed, using an amino acid (protein) powder for two meals a day. The third meal was to be a simple combination of hypoallergenic grains such as millet, rice, and vegetables. The purpose of this diet was to give his body a rest.

A variety of supplements were used, including coenzyme Q10, N-acetyl cysteine (an antiviral herbal substance), and gingko biloba (for increasing peripheral and micro circulation). A modest detoxification program was initiated with drinking lots of water and taking a flaxseed hull colon cleanser that absorbs toxins in the bowel. He was instructed to begin very light exercise in the form of walking outdoors daily in the fresh air.

After following this regime for two months he had improved to 65 percent of normal functioning, and at two years he described himself as back to 100 percent.

tions there is no specific conventional therapy or the effectiveness of the therapy is unknown.[9]

Historically, of course, naturopathic institutions have been outside the loop of research funding by government and the pharmaceutical and insurance industries. Still, recent years have seen a growing list of important contributions.

Recent Studies

A perusal of recently published studies from naturopathic colleges finds the following examples:

- antitumor activity of maitake mushrooms[10]
- absorption of various forms of zinc (zinc is now widely recognized as important for immunity and prevention of prostate cancer)[11]
- effects of garlic oil on blood clotting, blood fats, and blood pressure[12]
- treatment of intestinal candidiasis (yeast overgrowth) with acidophilus [13] and homeopathy[14]
- naturopathic treatment of HIV infection[15]
- naturopathic treatment of hematoma[16]
- clinical manifestations of HIV in women[17]
- cancer and nutritional therapy[18]
- physiological effects of colon hydrotherapy[19]
- herbal treatment of allergic rhinitis (sinus inflammation)[20]

Other projects currently underway or recently completed at naturopathic medical schools include:

- outcomes of patients undergoing alternative cancer therapy at three Mexican cancer clinics
- effect of vitamin E on cholesterol
- absorption of different forms of calcium
- allergenic properties of primitive wheat strains
- management of leiomyoma in premenopausal women
- a double-blind placebo-controlled trial on the effects of a homeopathic treatment on osteoarthritis of the knee
- the effects of a botanical formula on endocrine functioning in menopausal women
- shark cartilage in treatment of Kaposi's sarcoma
- a naturopathic treatment protocol for Giardia infection
- a naturopathic treatment protocol for weight loss and chronic diarrhea in AIDS patients

- naturopathic treatment protocols for cervical dysplasia (precancerous cells)
- participation in a nationwide ten-year study of the safety and efficacy of the cervical cap as a method of birth control
- clinical assessment of food sensitivities
- a clinical trial of odorless garlic in the treatment of candidiasis (yeast overgrowth) in multiple bodily systems
- effects of aloe vera on symptoms of migraine

With the growing demand for nontoxic therapies for serious illnesses, naturopathic research is gaining a higher profile. For example, Leanna Standish, N.D., Ph.D., research director at Bastyr University of Natural Health Sciences and an advisor to the Office of Alternative Medicine, National Institutes of Health, is examining naturopathic treatments in people with HIV. Using nutritional and herbal therapies, Standish has found improvement in some measures of immunity and a slower progression to AIDS compared to controls receiving only conventional therapy.[21]

Support from the Mainstream

A tremendous amount of scientific support for the principles of naturopathic medicine has been conducted at mainstream research centers. In fact, allopathy is increasingly turning to the use of natural methods in the search for effective treatments for today's intractable and expensive chronic diseases.

HIV. One of the most dramatic examples is the work of San Francisco physician Jon Kaiser, M.D., who has developed a program of diet, exercise, vitamins, herbs, and stress reduction that has shown promise in arresting the progression of AIDS. Kaiser's approach is to consider HIV not so much as an invader but as a potentially dormant virus like a herpes virus that can live in the system for years—perhaps one's entire lifetime—without causing symptoms.

Claire

Claire, a forty-five-year-old woman, sought help for dermatitis and an itchy skin rash. She also happened to have a condition called retinitis pigmentosa, a chronic degenerative eye disease that progressively leads to blindness. She could see vague shapes but had to be led into the office.

She was placed on a specific diet to remove foods for which she had intolerances, including eggs and potatoes, particularly when eaten in combination with grains. The naturopath also began a regime of hydrotherapy and gave her a homeopathic remedy (phosphorous).

After three weeks of hydrotherapy Claire reported she was beginning to see better. After six weeks her skin rash was gone, she could tell the color of the naturopath's eyes, could read large print books, and could walk into the office by herself.

According to Jared Zeff, N.D., L.Ac., "I learned from this case that there are no incurable diseases. The recuperative powers of the body are amazing and unpredictable. The real basis of the work is improving health, and as health improves, problems begin to disappear. Claire's vision never returned to normal but had improved to the point where she could read.

"This illustrates how as digestion improves and toxemia decreases, everything will start to improve if there is any potential for it to improve at all."

He believes that dormancy is an achievable phenomenon by creating an environment in the body that is inhospitable to HIV, "encouraging" the virus to remain dormant. Using his combination of natural therapies with a very modest use of allopathic drugs, 89 percent of 134 HIV positive patients in his

Pam

Pam is a forty-year-old real estate agent who had significant rheumatoid arthritis in her hands, wrists, and feet. She was just starting to use a synthetic anti-inflammatory drug.

She sought naturopathy because she was concerned about the side effects of the drug. Through a dietary assessment, pulse and tongue diagnosis, and palpation of the abdomen, the practitioner determined that she had a fruit intolerance. She was taken off fruit, her diet was adjusted in other ways (in naturopathic theory, the physical basis of the inflammation in arthritis is metabolic waste as a result of poor digestion), and she used daily hydrotherapy. She became progressively better each of the four succeeding weeks. One month later she had no more arthritis and reported feeling better than she ever had in her life.

practice have remained stable or improved their diagnosis during a five-year period.[22]

Heart Disease. Kaiser is practicing a good example of integrative medicine (as discussed in Chapter 10). Another case is the work of Dean Ornish, M.D., director of the Preventive Medicine Research Institute at the University of California, San Francisco. In a widely acclaimed study, Ornish found that patients with severe coronary heart disease could not only arrest but actually *reverse* their condition, something not previously thought possible in conventional medical circles, where expensive heart bypass surgery had become the rule (having increased 186 percent in the decade of the 1980s[23]).

Ornish's program consists of a very low-fat diet (with animal fats counting for less than 10 percent of total calories), stress management through meditation and yoga, moderate exercise, and participation in a weekly support group.[24] In addition, this obviously cost-effective treatment program (one tenth the cost of coronary bypass surgery) is now being covered by insurance companies as an alternative to expensive surgery and drugs.

Heart Attack. In a related study, researchers in the Netherlands found evidence that flavonoids, a natural substance found in apples, onions, and tea, may reduce the risk of death from coronary heart disease. Reported in the prestigious journal *The Lancet*, the five-year study of 805 Dutch men between the ages of sixty-five and eighty-four found that those who consumed the highest amounts of flavonoids suffered about half as many fatal heart attacks as those who consumed the lowest amounts.[25]

These results were independent of other risk factors such as high blood pressure, obesity, high cholesterol, and smoking. The men's highest source of flavonoids was tea, leading scientists to speculate that flavonoids might protect the heart by preventing the formation of plaque that clogs the arteries, by lowering cholesterol, or by lowering blood pressure.

In another study, Dr. JoAnn Manson of Harvard found that women with diets rich in vitamins A and C and beta carotene had a 33-percent lower risk of heart attacks and a 71-percent lower risk of strokes than women whose diets more nearly resembled the average intake of those vitamins.[26]

Arthritis. A promising new treatment for rheumatoid arthritis has been found in a natural substance, a form of a collagen solution made from chicken cartilage. Researchers at Harvard found that consuming this protein material, which is similar to the membrane of the joints being attacked by the immune system in this disorder, "reinstructs the body to cease the attack on the body's own joints." In a controlled clinical trial, all patients taking the cartilage substance got better, while most of those taking the placebo got worse.[27]

Prostate Cancer. Another compelling study demonstrates the wisdom of naturopathy's perennial nutritional guidelines about reducing consumption of red meat. A study conducted by researchers at Harvard and the Mayo Clinic of 47,000 men found that heavy consumption of animal fat, especially red meat, increases the risk of advanced life-threatening prostate cancer. Men who ate red meat five or more times a week were 2.6 times as likely to develop advanced prostate cancer as those who ate it once a week or less. The study found no link between prostate cancer and fat in poultry or diary.[28]

Colon Cancer. A Dutch study of 120,000 men and women found a 72-percent increase in colon cancer among those who ate more than twenty grams (seven-tenths of an ounce) of processed meat, such as sausages, per day.[29]

Dietary Therapy. These are a few examples of literally thousands of scientific studies, many of which are controlled and double-blind, on the effects of natural and dietary substances on health. There is now broad acceptance by even the most conservative mainstream institutions of the role of diet and nutrition in many illnesses. The American Cancer Society, the National Cancer Institute, and the American Heart Association all now make dietary recommendations.

One recent study at Johns Hopkins University found that a compound isolated from broccoli, called sulforaphane, blocks the growth of tumors in mice treated with a cancer-causing toxin. The substance is found in other cruciferous vegetables such as cauliflower, cabbage, and brussels sprouts.[30]

Recent reports have also noted that multivitamin supplementation delays the onset of AIDS in HIV positive individuals. And leading researchers of chronic fatigue immune dysfunction syndrome are now using vitamin and mineral supplementation to combat the effects of hypovitaminosis—nutritional deficiencies at the cellular level that impair the immune system's ability to heal itself.[31] It is ironic that, while therapeutic nutrition is at the heart of naturopathic medical education, few allopathic medical schools include such courses in their curricula.

According to Melvyn Werbach, M.D., assistant clinical professor at the UCLA School of Medicine, "It is now well estab-

Monica

Monica, an eight-year-old girl, had taken eight courses of antibiotics over the last five years for chronic ear infections. Surgical insertion of ear tubes was being considered.

She was taken off milk, given a homeopathic remedy, and had two weeks of hydrotherapy (alternating hot and cold packs to the trunk). She stopped having ear infections.

According to Jared Zeff, N.D., L.Ac., "Every case [of otitis media] I've seen has cleared up with dietary changes. Eighty percent of these kids have a milk intolerance.

"The hydrotherapy lowers the level of metabolic waste products in the blood by improving digestion and elimination. We can also use specific hydrotherapy. If the child wakes up during the night with pain in the ear, the parent can put cold wet socks on both the child's feet, cover them with wool socks, and give an acute homeopathic remedy (usually belladonna or pulsatilla). The hydrotherapy improves circulation to the ear by stimulating peripheral circulation throughout the body and in a sense pulls the inflammation out of the ear. Combined with homeopathy, the child will usually be asleep in about twenty minutes."

lished . . . that nutritional factors are of major importance in the pathogenesis of both atherosclerosis and cancer, the two leading causes of death in Western countries, and studies validating their importance in the pathogenesis of many other diseases continue to be published."[32]

For the professional, an excellent compilation of research is offered in Dr. Werbach's book *Nutritional Influences on Illness:*

Lucy

Lucy, a four-year-old girl, had developed a painful earache for two days. Her parents used the cold socks treatment: she soaked her feet in a tub of hot water for eight minutes, then put on a pair of cotton socks that had been soaked in cold water and wrung out, covered these with a pair of dry wool socks, and went straight to bed. In addition she took a homeopathic remedy (belladonna). Within thirty minutes she was asleep and when she awoke the next morning the earache was gone.

A Sourcebook of Clinical Research. This 620-page compendium presents abstracts of thousands of clinical studies on nutritional factors in eighty-seven conditions and diseases (e.g., atherosclerosis, mitral valve prolapse, candidiasis, scleroderma, prostatitis, and so on).[33] A similar volume entitled *Nutritional Influences on Mental Illness* is also available.[34]

For the layperson, three practical guides to research-based nutrition programs are Dr. Michael Murray's *The Healing Power of Foods* (Prima Publications, 1993), Dr. Elson Haas's *Staying Healthy with Nutrition* (Celestial Arts, 1991), and Werbach's *Healing through Nutrition* (HarperCollins, 1993).

Research on Cost-Effectiveness

One important area of research to naturopaths is cost-effectiveness. As a rule, any ailment that is successfully treated with natural means will be treated for much less than the cost of conventional drugs or other medical procedures. As noted earlier, the Ornish program for reversing heart disease cost about a tenth as much as conventional treatment.

As another example, a study of obstetric care provided by a sample of forty-three naturopathic physicians found the following: 1530 births were scheduled for home birth or birth in a clinic or birthing center. Eight percent were changed to hospital birth before labor due to risk factors and 7 percent were transferred to the hospital during labor due to complications.

Total cesarean-section rate of all patients, including those transferred to the hospital prior to labor due to increased risk, was 6 percent.[35] The normal c-section rate for conventional-style hospital deliveries is about 25 percent. C-section and other hospital births are of course substantially more expensive than home births or births in a birthing center. This illustrates what many proponents of naturopathy consider one of the most important benefits of this tradition, its savings in costly invasive procedures.

Another study compared relative costs of conventional drug treatment and dietary treatment for patients with elevated blood cholesterol. As could be expected, dietary treatment was found to be dramatically more cost-effective.[36]

In Germany, naturopathic services have been found so cost-effective that the government now requires conventional doctors and pharmacists to receive education in naturopathic methods and botanical medicine.

STRENGTHS AND LIMITATIONS

Naturopathy's best function is in primary care, general practice medicine with nontoxic, noninvasive methods. The greatest strengths are in preventive medicine, acute illnesses, and chronic illnesses that have not responded well to other medical traditions. Another strength is in natural childbirth, where the need for cesarean sections is much lower than in conventional care.

More than any other tradition, naturopaths excel in the area of clinical nutrition, with their command of research-based dietary protocols for a plethora of specific diseases. This is to be expected since this is a major emphasis in naturopathic medical education.

While naturopaths are trained in minor bone setting and X ray, they generally refer out to allopaths for broken bones. They are not trained in major surgery or acute trauma care. As stated by Zeff, "We can contribute to that, but we're not the primary person that puts the broken body back together. We can help with the healing process, but the M.D.s keep them alive and screw them back together, so to speak."

In many states it is illegal for practitioners from traditions other than allopathy to treat cancer. Hence, while naturopaths will work with cancer patients from the point of view of supporting their overall health and host resistance, they will not claim to be treating the disease. Such support can be of benefit, of course, for coping with the side effects of surgery, chemotherapy, and radiation, as well as strengthening overall host resistance. While many former cancer patients attribute their recoveries to natural methods, in the current legal climate it is not wise for naturopaths to claim credit for these outcomes.

THE PRACTITIONER-PATIENT RELATIONSHIP

Since this tradition focuses on the person rather than the diagnosis and treatment of disease entities, the training of naturopaths includes a great deal of preparation in counseling and communication skills. For example, the curriculum at National College of Naturopathic Medicine includes seven courses in this area. This is necessary because patient compliance and lifestyle modification play such a key role in many healing processes.

This puts the practitioner in the position of needing to cultivate a relationship with the patient in order to have influence on how that person lives outside the office. The role of teacher that naturopaths often take on is evident here, in that they will

Mel

Mel was suffering from reflux esophagitis, a crippling condition in which the valve at the top of the stomach does not close properly, resulting in extreme pain and discomfort in the esophagus.

A stool test found him to have a deficient level of stomach acid, a bacterial imbalance and candida in the colon, and no *E. coli* (a healthful form of intestinal bacteria).

He was given some friendly flora to restore the bacterial balance in his colon, some antifungal herbs for candida, short chain fatty acids, and licorice extract for his reflux esophagitis. He was also given digestive enzymes and some Chinese herbs to improve digestion.

His experiences of reflux diminished gradually over the next six months until they became quite rare.

help the patient develop realistic expectations for the benefits of following through with recommendations.

One of the by-products of this approach, of course, is that the doctor-patient relationship takes on a greater personal significance. Patients often feel a sense of interpersonal support and caring as a result. Some practitioners use telephone contact between visits to monitor progress and keep in touch with the patient.

EVALUATING PERSONAL RESULTS

Personal results are evaluated via the patient's subjective reports of changes in symptoms, the practitioner's observations, and laboratory tests when taken. In addition, depending on the modalities used, other means may be included such as pulse or tongue diagnosis. (See Chapters 2 and 3 on Chinese medicine and Ayurveda for explanation of these methods.)

RELATIONSHIP TO OTHER FORMS OF MEDICINE

Naturopaths view themselves as part of a broad, comprehensive, multitradition approach to health care. Thus they acknowledge the strengths and essential roles of other traditions. They view themselves as complementary and not exclusive of any other tradition. Often their methods can be used alongside other therapies in a supportive way.

Michael Murray, N.D., addresses this as follows: "I'm a pragmatist. I want the best thing for the patient. Sometimes that best thing is a blend of allopathic medicine and naturopathic medicine. I'm not an exclusionist by any means. I think 'complementary' is a good term for anyone involved in the healing professions. We all have our areas of expertise and experience."

Ironically, some of the greatest champions of naturopathic principles were originally trained in the allopathic tradition. For example, in addition to Dean Ornish, M.D., Melvyn Werbach, M.D., Jon Kaiser, M.D., and Elson Haas, M.D., other popular authorities include Andrew Weil, M.D., professor at the University of Arizona College of Medicine and author of *Natural Health, Natural Medicine* and *Spontaneous Healing*, and Robert Atkins, M.D., author of *Dr. Atkins' New Diet Revolution* and *Dr. Atkins' Health Revolution*.

Practitioners who were originally trained in other traditions and now use naturopathic principles often describe their work as "natural" medicine rather than "naturopathic" medicine.

COSTS

According to audits of naturopathic services and insurance company data, naturopathic office visits are about half as expensive as conventional medicine.[37] This does not include further cost savings that accrue as a result of the long-term preventive focus and the avoidance of more costly chronic illnesses. Reasons for the lower cost include substantially lower office overhead because of less emphasis on high-technology medical equipment and procedures, much lower malpractice insurance costs due to the extreme rarity of litigation, and other market forces.

In many cases naturopathic medicine offers inexpensive therapeutic alternatives to common medical procedures such as hysterectomy, prostate surgery, tonsillectomy, and other procedures that have been found to be frequently overused.

The cost of natural substances such as nutritional supplements and herbs is generally much lower than pharmaceutical drugs and such materials are usually available over the counter.

Insurance coverage varies by state and policy. Many companies will cover naturopathic medicine, and at least one uses naturopaths as gatekeeper physicians for patients seeking entry to health care services. In Connecticut naturopaths enjoy 100 percent coverage mandated by state law.

CHOOSING A PRACTITIONER

Training

There are three colleges in North America accredited by the Council on Naturopathic Medical Education (CNME): Bastyr University of Natural Health Sciences, Seattle, Washington; National College of Naturopathic Medicine, Portland, Oregon; and The Canadian College of Naturopathic Medicine, Toronto,

Ontario, Canada. A fourth, Southwest College of Naturopathic Medicine and Health Sciences in Scottsdale, Arizona, opened its doors in 1993 and at this writing is a candidate for accreditation. These are four-year programs that meet licensing requirements in those states and provinces that license naturopaths.

There are a few other programs that grant N.D. degrees that do not have standardized naturopathic curricula and do not meet accreditation guidelines. Some of these grant degrees are based on life experience or correspondence study, with no clinical training, and they are not recognized by licensing bodies. The lack of a uniform standard makes it more difficult for the consumer to evaluate the preparation of such practitioners.

Licensing

The legal status of naturopaths varies in different jurisdictions. Some states and provinces have specific laws and others do not, though they may allow naturopaths to practice to varying degrees. An increasing number of states are adopting a standard national exam (NPLEX—Naturopathic Physician Licensing Examination) as part of their credentialing process. The following states and provinces have specific licensing laws at this writing:

Alaska	Connecticut	Ontario
Alberta	Hawaii	Oregon
Arizona	Manitoba	Saskatchewan
British Columbia	Montana	Washington
	New Hampshire	

Right-to-practice laws exist in Idaho and North Carolina. Some naturopathic physicians are licensed to practice in Florida and Utah, though no new licenses have been issued for several years.

Paul

Paul had a chronic bladder infection with pain for four months. He had been through four courses of antibiotics. His allopathic physician suggested he be kept on the antibiotics indefinitely. He also reported headaches, back pain, and knee problems.

Paul sought a naturopath to see if there was another form of therapy available. The naturopath gave him a cleansing diet, a daily regime of hydrotherapy, and some herbs to soothe and clean the kidneys and bladder. He was given a Chinese herbal formula to strengthen the Kidney system and a Western herbal combination (a disinfectant—berberis and goldenseal). The next day the pain was much improved.

According to Jared Zeff, N.D., L.Ac., "He doesn't just have a bladder problem, he has a *pattern* of dysfunction. His digestion is not working the way it should so he's generating more metabolic waste products. The bacteria aren't the cause of the problem; they're living off the imbalance in his biochemistry. By normalizing diet and digestion, his biochemistry will improve and will no longer support a bacterial colony that shouldn't be there. His body, his urine, and his bladder had been a culture medium for the bacteria."

Zeff continues, "It's going to take another three or four weeks and the entire pattern of symptoms will improve."

Currently several states are in the process of considering legislation to establish licensure.

You may contact the AANP (see below) to determine the legal status of naturopathy in your state and to get a listing of qualified naturopaths.

Organizations

The American Association of Naturopathic Physicians (AANP) is the leading professional organization, with about 750 members, and is active in maintaining standards of practice, encouraging research, and supporting legislative efforts for proper regulation of practice. Most members are graduates of the three schools in North America that are accredited by the CNME. A few practitioners have been grandfathered in from defunct programs. The AANP publishes the *Journal of Naturopathic Medicine*, which includes original research and clinical practice articles. The organization also maintains a list to help consumers locate a naturopathic physician. Address: 2366 Eastlake Ave. E, Suite 322, Seattle, WA 98102, phone (206) 323-7610, FAX (206) 323-7612.

There are twenty-four state associations of naturopathic physicians.

The Homeopathic Academy of Naturopathic Physicians confers the title "Diplomate in the Homeopathic Academy of Naturopathic Physicians" (D.H.A.N.P.) based on a written and practical competency exam. They publish *Similimum*, a quarterly journal on classical homeopathy, and a directory of diplomates. Address: P.O. Box 69565, Portland, OR 97201, phone (503) 795-0579.

Council on Naturopathic Medical Education (CNME) was first recognized in 1987 by the U.S. Department of Education as the accrediting body for naturopathic medical colleges. Address: P.O. Box 11426, Eugene, OR 97440–3626, phone (503) 484–6028.

Canadian Naturopathic Association maintains a list of registered naturopaths in Canada. Address: P.O. Box 4520, Station C, Calgary, Alberta T2T 5N3, Canada, phone (403) 244–4487.

Conclusion

Beyond determining the practitioner's legal license status and whether they were trained in an accredited program, an important question is that of his or her specialization. You cannot assume that just because someone is a naturopath they are going to take a certain approach, because of the wide diversity in this tradition. If you feel drawn to the general philosophy of naturopathy, since it encompasses such a wide range of practices, you may want to consider what modalities feel right to you.

Aside from these considerations, we return to the issue of how personally comfortable you feel in the practitioner's presence. Do you feel a sense of respect and that there is reliable communication? As with any other tradition your ability to trust the practitioner is a key in creating a climate for healing.

CHAPTER 5

HOMEOPATHY: THE GRAND PROVOCATEUR

"The introduction of homeopathy forced the old school doctor to stir around and learn something of a rational nature about his business. You may honestly feel grateful that homeopathy survived the attempts of the allopathists [orthodox physicians] to destroy it."

—Mark Twain[1]

Homeopathy has been a significant part of American medicine since the turn of this century when about 15 percent of physicians were homeopaths. There were twenty-two homeopathic medical schools, including Boston University, University of Michigan, New York Medical College, University of Minnesota, and Hahnemann Medical College. In addition there were a hundred homeopathic hospitals and over a thousand homeopathic pharmacies.[2]

The profile of homeopathy became overshadowed, however, by the tremendous growth of conventional pharmaceutical medicine and the political and legislative advances of the allopathic tradition. This was spearheaded largely by the rise in prominence of the American Medical Association. In 1912, the American Institute of Homeopathy, the nation's oldest medical society, formally challenged the AMA to a controlled clinical trial to compare the effectiveness of homeopathy versus allopathic medicine, which the

AMA declined.[3] While allopathy became embedded as the predominant tradition in many of society's institutions, homeopathy continued to be practiced, though on a smaller scale.

One of the leading forces in the passage of the federal Food, Drug, and Cosmetics Act in 1938 was Senator Royal Copeland, a homeopathic physician from New York. Copeland had previously been dean of the New York Homeopathic Medical College (today known as New York Medical College) and also health commissioner of New York City.

This act created the Food and Drug Administration (FDA) and empowered it to define drugs as either over-the-counter (OTC) or requiring a prescription. Homeopathic medicines were included in the former category. OTC drugs have to be basically safe and are allowed to be accompanied by health claims for nonserious health problems and self-limiting conditions not requiring medical supervision. Homeopathic remedies can be clearly identified as, for example, for insomnia, arthritis, teething, or the like.

Today, homeopathy is undergoing a resurgence of popularity in the United States. Sales of homeopathic medicines grew by 1000 percent from the 1970s to the early 1980s[4] and by 50 percent between 1988 and 1990.[5] There are probably between one and two thousand homeopaths practicing in North America, including five hundred physicians.[6] A 1993 report in *The New England Journal of Medicine* suggested that 2.5 million Americans used homeopathic medicines and 800,000 patients visited homeopaths in 1990.[7]

KEY PRINCIPLES

The Law of Similars

Homeopathy traces its roots to Hippocrates, who taught 2400 years ago about the law of similars. This once obscure principle was rediscovered in the 1790s by the German physician Samuel Hahnemann. Through experimentation on himself, Hahnemann found that Peruvian bark, which contains quinine and was used to treat malaria, caused malaria-like symptoms if taken when there was no malaria. He then began experimenting with other substances and so began a tradition of accumulated clinical experimentation.

Hahnemann found that other materials from plants, animals, and minerals could also cure the same symptoms they would cause. The essence of the law of similars is like cures like, in which the first "like" refers to the *substance* that would cause a certain set of symptoms in a healthy person and the second "like" refers to those same symptoms when present in an ill person.

Remedies

The remedies are drawn from nature, including herbs, animal products, and minerals. They are usually administered in the form of small pills that enter the bloodstream directly by dissolving under the tongue. They are prepared by a process called potentization, which involves repeatedly diluting and shaking the material until only an extremely dilute amount remains.

A remedy may go through two hundred or more cycles of being further diluted and shaken. The theory holds that the more dilute a remedy is, the longer it will act, the deeper will be the effect, and the fewer doses will be needed. Practitioners have approximately two thousand remedies available from which to choose. Each remedy has been experimentally tested on human beings to determine what types of individuals respond most strongly to the substances.

One of the great mysteries of homeopathy is that the dilution of these substances, or potentization to nearly infinitesimally small amounts, can have such beneficial effects against their associated symptoms. Yet remedies are often diluted to such a degree that *there are no remaining molecules of the original tincture present in the remedy.*

Since it is apparently not the chemistry, in the molecular sense, of the substance that has an effect on the person, it must be something else. That "something else" is perhaps what Dana Ullman, M.P.H., calls a "holographic imprint" of some energetic aspect of the substance. The subtle energetic qualities of the original substance are somehow acting upon the energetic qualities of the person.

The Vital Force

Hahnemann postulated that people have a vital force that is being influenced. He asserted that the vital force is the organizing, enlivening energy that keeps us healthy. Since it is this vital force that is affected by the energetic qualities of the remedies, homeopathy is often referred to as a form of energetic medicine. We are using one subtle energy, that of the remedy, to influence another energy, the energy field of the person or vital force, to raise itself to a higher degree of organization or functioning, thereby eliminating symptoms that have occurred in the body.

"Vital force" is a concept somewhat similar to that of *chi* in Chinese medicine or *prana* in Ayurveda. Western science has no parallel concept. As Hahnemann observed, when symptoms of illness occur, this vital force can be aroused to a higher level, thereby helping the body to use its own inner resources to alleviate the symptoms.

Here is where homeopathy differs dramatically from the thinking of other traditions. The remedies are not selected to *support* the nutritional or metabolic needs of the body nor to attack pathogens. Rather, the goal is to very subtly *provoke* or *challenge* the vital force, in a sense arousing it so that it will bring all the body's systems to a higher level of order and harmony, thereby eliminating the symptoms and pathogens.

Types of Remedies

There are three broad types of remedies: *acute*, *chronic*, and *constitutional*. An acute remedy is one given for an acute set of symptoms in which a more prompt response is needed. An example is for flu, where people have fever, achiness, sore throat, and so on. Research has shown that flu patients recover much faster when given such a remedy.[8] In acute diseases, relief can come anywhere from a few hours to a day or two following a remedy.

A chronic remedy is given for more long-standing problems and it is expected that the length of time for a cure is determined in part by how long the person has had the symptoms. Relief may take as much as three months to two years.

After a person has recovered from acute or chronic symptoms, a constitutional remedy may be given to strengthen their resistance to developing symptoms in the future. The constitutional remedy works more slowly and works to strengthen the body in a more diffuse way. It is the one remedy that addresses all the patient's symptoms, vulnerabilities, and unique personality and genetic characteristics. In many cases, an acute or chronic remedy may also serve as a constitutional remedy.

The Role of Symptoms

In diagnosis, the homeopath is not focusing on a conventional medical diagnosis, but rather on gleaning an accurate picture of the symptoms themselves. The symptom picture is then matched with a remedy. The ideal remedy is the one substance that would create the exact same symptom pattern if given to a healthy person. By doing this, a generalized defense response is triggered in which the whole organism functions in a better way, both physically and mentally.

In this tradition symptoms are considered efforts of the body to adapt and restore balance or homeostasis in the face of an infection or other stress on the body. Treatment is thus an attempt to provoke the body to summon up its own healing resources rather than having the treatment itself alleviate the symptoms.

Seemingly unrelated symptoms, occurring on many levels, are treated together. According to Nancy Herrick, N.P., of the Hahnemann Clinic in Albany, California, "The remedies stimulate a deep cure on emotional, mental, as well as physical levels of the person. It's a very profound response if you get the correct remedy. It can cure long, deeply held phobias, for example, as well as chronic diarrhea. In other words, if we select the right remedy, however we manage to select it, it will cure that person on all levels."

This is a highly individualized treatment in that two people with the same disease may have unique patterns in how their symptoms manifest. The focus is on treating according to the patient's responses rather than according to the cause of the disease. This presents, in a sense, an advantage over allopathic medicine, in that the cause of the disease need not be known in order to treat the patient.

Proponents also believe that modern technological and pharmaceutical medicine carries risks of unknown long-term effects on people. The argument is that these modern interventions do not work by strengthening people, but may actually be interfering with the body's own efforts to heal by artificially suppressing the symptoms. Such treatment may ultimately weaken the vital force.

In this view, what is needed in an instance of illness is for the person's vital force to be stronger, and not necessarily the introduction of some outside agent to destroy a pathogen. Again, the symptoms are considered a by-product of the organism's efforts to heal.

Homeopaths point to the overuse of pharmaceutical drugs as a major factor in our overall decline of health. For example, according to Michael Carlston, M.D., D.Ht., assistant clinical professor of family and community medicine at the University of California, San Francisco, "It's very clear in my mind that

Curing Asthma

A thirty-six-year-old physician sought help for asthma of eighteen years' duration. He had been taking three kinds of asthma medication concurrently since high school. He was given a constitutional remedy to take daily. His symptoms gradually diminished until he was able to discontinue one medication, then the second, and finally the third. At eighteen months he discontinued the homeopathic treatment and was symptom-free. He was seen for a total of four sessions.

recurrent ear infections in kids are a result of the antibiotics that are used. Out of two to three hundred new kids per year with recurrent ear infections, I see maybe two who aren't helped by homeopathy. And that's better than surgery is. Part of it is putting the brakes on the cycle of giving them antibiotics all the time. They can be used selectively, but if you can get better in other ways, it makes a lot more sense."

Antidoting

Antidotes are substances whose qualities are thought capable of destroying the beneficial action of a remedy. These include coffee, camphor, mint, other strong tastes or scents, many prescription or recreational drugs, electric blankets, and even dental drilling.

Homeopathic experts disagree about how important a consideration this is. Most believe that certain substances must be avoided, at least for a short length of time, after which the cure is permanent and will be unaffected by them. Others are convinced that if truly the right remedy is selected, then antidoting is not a concern in the first place.

This may be a matter of individual differences, at least to some degree, in that some people may be antidoted by a certain substance while others may not be. According to Roger Morrison, M.D., also of the Hahnemann Clinic, coffee will antidote about two-thirds of people, but it is impossible to predict who will be affected.

He describes a case in which a person who had been treated for asthma was symptom-free for a year. Upon drinking a cup of coffee, all the symptoms returned. In another case, a child was treated successfully for terrible migraine headaches. Five years later, she had her teeth drilled on and the next day her migraine headaches returned.

Herrick tells of another child who had been successfully treated for severe migraines. Her mother accidentally put some coffee in some pancake batter, and as the child was eating them the headaches returned.

On the other hand, Carlston describes a case of a patient who was wheelchair-bound with MS. "I gave him a remedy, and he came back after a year just to show me how good he was. He was walking without a cane. He drinks two cups of coffee a day." He describes another case of a woman who had had a psychotic break and is now doing fine, also drinking two cups a day.

According to Carlston, the challenge to the practitioner is finding the right remedy. Some are more right than others, and the more right the choice of remedy, the less vulnerable it is to being antidoted. "I feel very doubtful that there's much that can really antidote [the right] remedy. At this point I warn people about a few things: dental drilling, coffee, electric blankets, camphor on the skin, and MRIs.

"But I've grown to be suspicious about all these things because people don't comply. They'll say, 'Oh, I only drink a cup of coffee a day, and I've been okay,' and I say 'Okay, fine, you can drink it.' What I say to my patients, once they've responded and are better, is if they want coffee, 'Go ahead and try it and let's see what happens.' "

The experience of the practitioner can be an important factor.

As Carlston states, "When you're new to homeopathy, you tend to think that you're giving people the right remedy, and if they get worse, you think they interfered with it. I find, especially in patients who have been treated by other homeopaths that said, 'Oh, you antidoted it,' that they missed the remedy. I may give a different remedy and they're fine."

How long a person must abstain from antidoting substances is unknown and could vary from six months to several years, perhaps depending in part on how long the person had the original illness. Ultimately, however, cures are thought to be indelible and antidoting is no longer a concern.

The Healing Process

In homeopathic theory, the more rapid the onset of the disease process, the more rapid the cure will be. A flu that has come on very suddenly will go away very suddenly, whereas a headache condition that has been chronic for several years will go away more slowly.

Homeopaths also pay attention to the sequence in which symptoms abate. Symptoms that are less severe are expected to diminish before the deeper symptoms or pathologies disappear.

For example, according to Herrick, "You may see an improvement on the emotional level and you know it's going to work more on the physical as time goes on. So the patient may say, 'I still have my ulcer, but I'm much more cheerful, my energy's better,' so you know the remedy's right. It's just a matter of waiting a little longer." On the other hand, if the ulcer had gone away first and the emotional problems remained, this might be an indication that the wrong remedy was used and a better choice was needed.

Often there is a healing crisis within a few days to a week or two following a remedy. This is a brief period in which symptoms may temporarily increase before they are relieved. This is a sign that the remedy is working and that the body has been successfully provoked to a higher level of healing responses.

Kevin

Kevin was a forty-four-year-old occupational safety consultant who had been suffering from migraine headaches, which had been getting worse each year for twenty years. He also had frequent sinus infections and low-level depression. He was treated with a variety of conventional medications for migraines. He was given one dose of *natrum muriaticum* and his migraines stopped that week. He had a total of two visits to the homeopath.

According to Herrick, remedies can have a profound effect on the emotional level. "Sometimes people may come just for the emotional state—for example, where they feel severe depression, where they feel like they're blocked and can't relate to people, they're locked in. And the remedy will help that emotional state dramatically." She describes the case of a very well-known professor, forty-five years old, at the top of his field, with severe depression:

He was referred by a psychotherapist and had suicidal tendencies, which he kept to himself. He had a tendency to use drugs and alcohol to keep himself up. We have a remedy, *aurum metallicum*, which is gold, that we use very often for heart disease. This remedy is one that has the sense of the heart encased in steel, in an emotional as well as a physical sense.

I gave him *aurum metallicum*. After the remedy, he was much more open to talking to his family. And then he just came back and said, "I'm better. I feel much better. The depression is much better, I'm much more able to talk and share what's going on with me, I'm much more effective in my work." I saw him twice after the initial interview for follow-up, six weeks later, and then six months later.

Prevention

Theoretically, if a person is well and has no symptoms, the homeopath has no basis on which to treat. Hence, it would not be possible to strengthen your vital force in anticipation of, say, an overseas trip to a third-world country. The homeopath may recommend herbs or nutritional supplements that other traditions might use for strengthening resistance, but no remedies would be indicated.

On the other hand, according to Carlston, "It's real important to stress that symptoms can be very subtle, and though the person may claim no symptoms, we may find there are subtle patterns that they don't perceive as problematic. . . . I see somebody pacing, and they say, 'I'm fine,' and then I'll say, 'You seem kind of anxious,' and I'll ask if they tend to be irritable when driving, and they'll say, 'Oh yeah, I can't stand being in line,' and then I'll give them a remedy."

This would be a constitutional remedy for fine-tuning the person's vital force. It would not be like building up reserves of a certain nutrient in the person's tissues. But in this sense, homeopathy can be thought of as preventive if such treatment helps the person resist other more serious illness.

VARIATIONS WITHIN THE TRADITION

Classical Homeopathy

Classical homeopaths are distinguished from the nonclassical by their interest in identifying and using constitutional remedies. These are based on an in-depth interview to understand all the patient's idiosyncratic symptoms in response to an illness, as well as their psychological, emotional, physical, and hereditary characteristics. The classical practitioner is interested in the person's unique pattern of symptoms in response to what may be a common ailment.

In order to make such an in-depth assessment of the person's symptom picture, an intimate knowledge of that person on all levels needs to be taken into account. This requires an investment of time in getting to know the patient well, usually a one- to two-hour initial consultation. This is distinguished from a nonclassical practitioner, who might arbitrarily give a certain remedy to everyone with a given ailment.

A classical homeopath adheres most closely to Hahnemann's principle of like cures like and does not prescribe on the basis of simply the illness alone, recognizing that different people with the same illness have different symptoms based on their own unique constitution. In addition to constitutional remedies, classical practitioners also use acute and chronic remedies.

Single-Remedy Homeopathy. This term applies to a variation of classical homeopathy that does not treat chronic underlying states, only acute conditions. Single remedies are commonly available in health food stores but are designated only by the name of the substance, e.g., pulsatilla. You have to know exactly what remedy is right for you, either upon recommendation of a practitioner or from your own study and experience, in order to use these effectively.

Often people use popular homeopathic guidebooks or first aid manuals that describe remedies in order to make these choices. Examples are: *Everybody's Guide to Homeopathic Medicines*, by Stephen Cummings, M.D., and Dana Ullman, M.P.H. (Los Angeles: Tarcher, 1991); *Homeopathic Medicine at Home*, by M. Panos, M.D., and Jane Heimlich (Tarcher, 1980); and *Homeopathic Medicine for Children and Infants*, by Dana Ullman, M.P.H. (Tarcher, 1992).

Lynnette

A nineteen-year-old university student, Lynnette had been suffering from severe rheumatoid arthritis for six months. She was taking systemic anti-inflammatory medication and other conventional medications and her condition seemed to be worsening. She was also on antidepressants to treat her depression.

She worked with a homeopath over a two-year period using two different remedies. Her symptoms gradually diminished to where she averaged one aspirin a week and no other medications. At one point she had a bout of smoking marijuana, which apparently antidoted her remedy, and the symptoms returned. She was given another dose and symptoms began to remit again.

She stopped taking the homeopathic remedy after two years and was free of both the rheumatoid arthritis and depressive symptoms. She had a total of six office visits to her homeopath over the two-year period.

Nonclassical Homeopathy

In this approach, the selection of remedies is not based on a detailed assessment of the person's unique constitution, age, or other differences. Rather, remedies are given based primarily on the ailment—acute or chronic. Everyone with a given condition will receive the same remedy. The term "nonclassical" applies to many health care practitioners from other traditions using homeopathic substances as well as to the practice of self-prescribing by the layperson who chooses a remedy at the health food store.

Formula or Combination Homeopathy. This involves the combining of several remedies that are thought by their manufacturers to be commonly effective for the widest range of people. There might be two to eight different substances mixed together, with the assumption that one of the components is likely to be right for the individual who is taking them—a sort of shotgun approach.

The combinations are usually named for the ailment they are intended to address, for example, Arthritis Pain, Cold and Flu, Dry Cough, Insomnia, Colic, Earache, Teething, Vaginitis, Sinusitis, Tension Headache, Migraine Headache, and so on.

Combination homeopathy is considered safe and sometimes effective for the more minor health problems but is rarely effective for more serious chronic conditions. Classical homeopaths tend to frown on this approach, with the concern that even if the right remedy is included in this mix, its effectiveness will be hampered by the presence of the other ones. Further, if a person tries a combination remedy and does not respond, which is not uncommon, they may reject homeopathy altogether. This can also happen with classical homeopathy, as no method of medicine is always effective.

Isopathy. The practice of isopathy is treating something with itself. The choice of a remedy is made based on the offending substance that *caused* symptoms in the person, not the person's unique constellation of responses to that substance. For example, a practitioner may give potentized thyroid to a person with thyroid problems. Or they might give a person with a bee sting *apis*, which is made from the honeybee. To the classical homeopath, these remedies are expected to be effective only 20 to 30 percent of the time because they do not fully take into account the person's unique constitution.

PROCEDURES AND TECHNIQUES

Classical Homeopathy

Before the first interview, many practitioners use a written questionnaire to gain an overall view of the person's medical history and current symptoms.

The initial interview may be followed in succeeding weeks with briefer interviews of fifteen to thirty minutes. The ideal most classical homeopaths strive for is the one-shot cure, though this is not always achieved. In the case of the classical homeopath, this involves an exhaustive, thorough interview in which the patient's symptom picture is understood within the context of their unique psychological, spiritual, emotional, behavioral, and physical aspects.

A single remedy is then prescribed that would be expected to create the same symptom picture in a person who has these same qualities. Theoretically, if the correct remedy is selected, it will change their entire system and all symptoms.

A third to half the interview may be devoted to the person's psychological characteristics. This is not out of a belief that the mind causes the symptoms, but rather that symptom complexes also manifest on the psychological level. In homeopathy there is a reciprocal interaction between body and mind. This also helps the practitioner to assess the person's history, constitutional state of health, and idiosyncratic symptoms.

The remedies are designed to enter the body's blood system through the mucus membranes of the mouth. The remedy usually comes in the form of either a tablet or small pellets that are absorbed under the tongue or liquid drops. You are cautioned not to consume any food or beverages or brush your teeth for at least fifteen minutes before and after taking a remedy. Also, it must not be touched by hands or fingers before contacting the mouth. In some cases, there may be daily doses the person will take during the course of an evaluation period.

Typically, the patient will be seen again in six weeks to two

148

months after the initial visit for evaluation. If progress has occurred, no additional remedy is given. They may be seen again in four to six months.

While the ideal for which practitioners strive is the single, one-shot cure, realistically this depends on getting the right remedy the first time. This is largely a matter of the skill and experience of the practitioner. Even the most skilled do not always get it right the first time. Practitioners are assisted by reference books filled with descriptions of remedies as well as by computer databases that help in describing remedies. Many practitioners will refer to their computer screen during the course of the interview for help in finding a remedy.

Often there is a trial period of two or three remedies and sometimes more before the right one is found. And in some cases it is never found. According to Morrison, "A competent homeopath should get the right remedy about 80 percent of the time by the second interview."

Laboratory testing, though not a part of homeopathic practice per se, is sometimes used to help establish a diagnosis—mainly to determine the severity of illness or to identify what particular illness the person has. This can help in establishing expectations as to how long it might take for progress to occur. Such tests are used much less than in conventional Western medicine, but they are used. A survey conducted by The American Institute of Homeopathy found the frequency of diagnostic testing was less than half that of allopathy (30 percent versus 68.5 percent).[9] This is a result of the fact that in homeopathy treatment is not determined by diagnosis but rather by symptoms.

Nonclassical Homeopathy

Remedies are often given in the context of treatment by other medical traditions. Many practitioners of allopathy, Chinese medicine, osteopathy, chiropractic, naturopathy, and Ayurveda use homeopathic substances, though some have been trained

149

classically and some have not. Usually they are taking the single-remedy approach in conjunction with the other modalities they offer in their routine practice. The more their homeopathic training is specialized, the better.

SCIENTIFIC SUPPORT

Medical historians believe that research on homeopathic substances marked the first use of clinical trials in medicine. This work began in the 1790s and continues today with fifteen to twenty substances currently being studied in various settings. There are just over two thousand remedies currently included in the homeopathic armamentarium, with over four thousand substances having been tested.

The method of testing remedies is called *proving* and is a process in which healthy people are given a substance to see what symptoms it causes. If there is a common pattern to the symptoms in the group, then the substance is considered proved for that pattern of symptoms. Further, the individuals being tested are each followed over a period of time to discern individual differences in how the substance affects people.

In order for a substance to be logged into the homeopathic literature as effective for a particular symptom, it has to cure the symptom multiple times. In other words, it not only has to produce the symptoms in healthy people, but it has to cure them in sick people.

The reference books and computer databases to which the homeopath turns in seeking a cure describe the symptoms observed in the proving of each remedy. Given the large number of remedies from which to choose, homeopaths believe that they should be able to find something that helps every single patient significantly.

Many of the substances were proven in sophisticated single- and double-blind scientific studies with large numbers of healthy people. Also, some substances were studied over several years or even several generations so the description of their actions

OAM-Funded Study

Michael Goldstein of the University of California, Los Angeles, has been funded to study the course of health for 130 new patients of three independent practitioners of classical homeopathy. The patients are followed for a period of four months from their initial entry into homeopathic treatment.

Questionnaires and extensive interviews are used to assess their medical status, quality of life, and beliefs about medicine. The goals include helping to determine which kinds of problems seem most responsive to classical homeopathy, what kinds of people do best with this tradition, and how its effectiveness can be best measured in future studies.

has been refined. In this sense, the entire practice of homeopathy is based on the scientific method.

Controlled Clinical Trials

There are some difficult challenges in designing good clinical trials of homeopathy that are not present in some other traditions. The main challenge is in choosing which kind of homeopathy to study: classical or combination. Clinical trials have been conducted with each of these distinctly different forms of homeopathy. Unfortunately, results are often used to support or condemn homeopathy in general rather than as evidence for the specific kind of homeopathy being studied.

Another challenge is that in those studies that focus on classical homeopathy, the skill of the practitioner is critical. If positive results are found, this would tend to support the principles of homeopathic treatment. But if negative results are found, how do we know whether this reflects on homeopathic principles or on the skill level of the practitioner who chose the remedies? Classical homeopaths would argue, of course, that negative findings may be attributed to the wrong remedies being used. This will likely be an ongoing source of debate in homeopathic research and is similar to the struggles encountered in acupuncture research, which is also a highly individualized skill-oriented form of intervention.

In an example of a study of classical homeopathy, a double-blind prospective study was conducted for homeopathic treatment of patients with rheumatoid arthritis. Over a three-month period, each patient received an individualized remedy while continuing with their ordinary anti-inflammatory medication. Patients treated with homeopathy were significantly improved over placebo controls (those receiving only conventional medication) in articular index, limbering-up time, grip strength, visual analog pain scale, and functional index.[10]

In a controlled double-blind study published in the journal *Pediatrics*, homeopathic remedies were used to treat acute diarrhea in eighty-one Nicaraguan children, ages six months to five years. Acute diarrhea is the world's leading cause of disease and death in children. The study was conducted by Dr. Jennifer Jacobs and her colleagues from the University of Washington School of Public Health and Community Medicine.

All children in the study received the usual oral hydration therapy. However, those who also received an individualized homeopathic remedy recovered significantly more quickly than those who received a placebo.[11]

A well-designed study of single-remedy homeopathy was done with a group of 487 patients with an influenzalike syndrome. Patients treated with a single remedy that was not individualized were 70 percent more likely to have recovered within forty-eight hours than those receiving the placebo. They also required less medication for symptoms and subjectively believed their treatment to be effective.[12]

Another controlled study, published in the prestigious journal

The Lancet, examined treatment of hay fever with a homeopathic preparation of mixed pollens. Allergic symptoms were
significantly reduced.[13]

These results were affirmed by yet another controlled study
published in *The Lancet* by a team of researchers from the
University of Glasgow. Twenty-eight patients with allergic
asthma were randomly assigned to either the experimental
group or the placebo group. Those receiving the homeopathic
remedy had significantly reduced symptoms and better respiratory functioning over the next eight weeks compared to those
receiving the placebo.[14]

A final example is a study of homeopathic treatment of fibromyalgia (a condition involving chronic muscle aches and
pains throughout the body). While this study used a single remedy for all patients, it adhered to classical homeopathic principles by selecting only patients whom the researcher determined
would warrant the same remedy based on their individual interviews. Each patient received the same medication for one month
and then a placebo for one month in random sequence. Highly
significant findings were the reduction of tender spots and improved relief from pain or ability to sleep, which are major
symptoms of this disorder.[15]

In early 1991, the *British Medical Journal* published a metanalysis of 107 controlled trials of the various forms of homeopathy
that took place between 1966 and 1990.[16] A metanalysis is a
technique of studying the outcomes of a large group of studies to
find overall trends in the research. Eighty-one of the studies showed
at least some degree of clinical benefits. The authors of the review,
who were two Dutch medical school professors and not homeopaths, reported: "The amount of positive evidence even among
the best studies came as a surprise to us. . . . The evidence presented
in this review would probably be sufficient for establishing homeopathy as a regular treatment for certain indications. . . ." Following is a summary of the results of their analysis:

• Four of nine trials showed benefits for vascular diseases.
• Thirteen of nineteen trials showed successful treatment of
  respiratory infections.

- Six of seven trials showed positive results in treating other infections.
- Five of seven trials showed improvement in diseases of the digestive system.
- Five of five trials showed successful treatment of hay fever.
- Five of seven trials showed faster recovery of bowel function after abdominal surgery.
- Four of six trials showed improvement in rheumatological disease.
- Eighteen of twenty trials found positive results in treating pain or trauma.
- Eight of ten trials showed positive results with mental or psychological problems.
- Thirteen of fifteen trials showed benefits for a variety of other conditions (duration and complications of delivery, diabetes, gas poisoning, myopia, cramps, lymphedema, respiratory insufficiency, and skin diseases).

One difficulty the scientific community has in accepting evidence for homeopathy's effects is that the mechanisms of how those effects are achieved are unknown. While it is believed that the effects are the result of some kind of electromagnetic or energetic influence of the remedies on the vital force, this is not well understood at this time, especially in Western scientific terms. Researchers are left with the uncomfortable question of whether we should accept a form of medicine whose mechanisms we do not understand, even if it has beneficial results.

This is precisely the question raised by the authors of the metanalysis described above, who asked, "Are the results of randomized double-blind trials convincing only if there is a plausible mechanism of action?" Debate continues over whether such understanding is needed in order to accept homeopathy or whether there is simply a widespread bias against this tradition because it represents a challenge to our conventional ways of thinking about health and healing.

For a further discussion of research and contemporary understanding of homeopathy, see *The Consumer's Guide to Homeopathy* by Dana Ullman, M.P.H. (New York: Tarcher/Putnam,

Adrienne

Adrienne, a thirty-eight-year-old bookkeeper, suffered from anxiety attacks and insomnia for eight months since having a root canal. She regularly used sleep medication and tranquilizers. She was given a homeopathic remedy, which she took daily in liquid form for ten months. Initially her symptoms were more severe for the first week and then gradually diminished until she dropped all medication at ten months. She had a total of four office visits.

1996) and *Homeopathy: A Frontier in Medical Science* by Paolo Bellavite, M.D., and Andrea Signorini, M.D. (Berkeley: North Atlantic, 1995).

STRENGTHS AND LIMITATIONS

In addition to the clinical research findings discussed above, proponents state that homeopathy is able to treat anything capable of being helped by the patient's own host resistance (natural defenses) or vital force. Obviously, it does not treat broken bones, although it may be used to speed the healing process once the bone is set. Homeopathy is also not generally considered a form of treatment for advanced cancer or advanced stages of other diseases, such as long-standing arthritis. It cannot repair a defective valve in the heart or stroke damage to the brain.

Its strengths lie in treatment of acute and chronic illnesses, particularly in the earlier stages or where there is not severe tissue damage. Migraine and headache conditions, as well as immune-related illnesses such as allergies or autoimmune diseases are often treated successfully with homeopathy, as are many chronic viral and bacterial infections.

Through its history homeopathy has been considered particularly effective with children. For example, Morrison reinforces some of Carlston's earlier comments by stating, "A child with an ear infection can be screaming and screaming, and you can put the right remedy on the child's tongue, and it's like somebody turned a radio off. They just go click, stop within two to three seconds, and may go to sleep right there, and then they wake up better. . . . The inflammation will be cut down almost instantaneously sometimes. And then suddenly the organism will mount a tremendous defense response and just clean up the infection." According to Herrick, children react very quickly because their systems are so pure.

Other children's ailments commonly treated include croup, acute diarrheas, bladder infections, teething problems, hyperactivity, emotional problems, behavior problems, and even learning disabilities, though the latter may take several months to respond. Seemingly spectacular anecdotal reports abound for many of these conditions. On the other hand, however, there are also cases where homeopathy has not helped for the same conditions, as evidenced by the story of Rose (see page 165). This underscores the nagging problem of inconsistency or unpredictability with some illnesses.

Herpes conditions are treated in large numbers by homeopaths and often respond dramatically, both in frequency and severity of attacks. According to Morrison, homeopathy is much more effective than Zovirax for herpes. "We'll have equivalent or sometimes superior response without any long-term side effects, whereas with long-term use of Zovirax, it's unsure how clinically safe it is."

Because of legal constraints, homeopathy is not used to treat cancer, syphilis, or gonorrhea. However, a homeopath who is also licensed to practice Western medicine may combine the two traditions, using homeopathic remedies along with the legally required drugs. In the case of cancer, for example, assuming the patient has been receiving the standard treatment of chemotherapy, radiation, or surgery, the homeopath may work to help

---

Scott

A forty-seven-year-old chiropractor, Scott had been suffering from severe depression, angry outbursts, low self-esteem, and low energy, which he described as a lifetime pattern of symptoms. He was given a single dose of a constitutional remedy and reported his symptoms had diminished 50 percent in the first week. His symptoms returned in three months, with his remedy apparently antidoted by coffee. He was given another dose and his symptoms disappeared.

---

strengthen the person's overall host resistance. They can also be treated for the nausea caused by the chemotherapy.

With regard to heart disease, the homeopathic literature reports many anecdotal cases in which certain heart diseases have responded well, including coronary artery disease, cardiac rhythm disturbances, and even cardiac failure.

Because of its symptom orientation, homeopathy is particularly important for people with conditions that conventional medicine has difficulty treating but that have unusual symptoms. Homeopaths find those kinds of people easier to treat, because their idiosyncratic symptoms help in making a clearer selection of remedies.

Homeopathy is often of value for pregnant and lactating women because it is widely recognized that they should avoid drugs, which can be passed on to infants. Homeopaths also believe that children should avoid drugs if possible, based on the idea that drugs are generally tested on adults and children's bodies respond differently than adults', which raises questions about safe dosages and long-term developmental effects.

Surprisingly, homeopathy actually gained its greatest popularity in Europe and America in the 1800s because of its successes in treating the infectious diseases of that era, including yellow fever, scarlet fever, cholera, and others. The death rates for some of these diseases were one-half to one-eighth those in conventional medical hospitals.[17,18] Hence, although conventional Western medicine today thinks of itself as very good in treating infectious diseases, and certainly is in some ways, so is homeopathy.

Finally, a strength of homeopathy is its lack of side effects. Since the remedies are given in such minute doses, there is not enough of the substance to cause toxic reactions or side effects in the body, as often happens with conventional drugs.

THE PRACTITIONER-PATIENT RELATIONSHIP

One of the hallmarks of classical homeopathy is the long, in-depth initial interview. However, while homeopaths would agree that the phenomenon of interpersonal caring is an important part of practice, this is not thought of as a key part of the healing equation. The real healing effects are attributed to the remedies themselves. The practitioner him or herself is not viewed so much as a healer as a skilled diagnostician and pre-scriber. The whole practice boils down to the technical process of finding the right remedy, though having good rapport and a sense of caring make this a more comfortable experience.

EVALUATING PERSONAL RESULTS

The patient's self-report with regard to symptoms is the main criterion of success. Patient and practitioner discuss this to-gether, and the practitioner's observations of change may also be part of this discussion.

While lab tests may be used in the initial diagnosis, they are generally not used to determine whether a remedy is working.

Again, this is a symptom-focused form of medicine and changes in the symptoms are the criteria of concern.

RELATIONSHIP TO OTHER FORMS OF MEDICINE

Homeopathy is used a great deal by practitioners who are grounded in other traditions. For example, in naturopathic medical education, homeopathy is one of the most popular majors or specialties after the student has completed basic science requirements. Their clinical training often involves working in clinics using homeopathic medicines as one of their primary therapeutic modes.

Practitioners tend to be less concerned about other traditions that use more natural forms of intervention, such as herbal or nutritional therapies, massage and bodywork, or mind/body medicine. However, acupuncture is considered an antidoting threat in some cases.

The question of using homeopathy with allopathic drugs is complicated by the issue of antidoting. Most practitioners would prefer that the person refrain from taking any other medication while undergoing homeopathic treatment. However, in some cases this is impossible, as, for example, in dilantin for epilepsy.

In the homeopathic perspective, allopathic drugs are designed to remove or suppress specific symptoms, which may interfere with remedies.

One strategy of getting around this is to give the remedy every day. Another is that the practitioner may carefully evaluate the seriousness of the need for the other medication, and if possible, wean the person from it gradually as the remedy is introduced. In this way, when it is apparent that the person is doing better without the other medication, they would hope to gradually discontinue it. Sometimes, however, the risks of discontinuing a drug may be deemed too great, in which case the person would simply not be a good candidate for homeopathic treatment.

COSTS

The initial interview with the classical homeopath may range from $100 to $400, depending on whether the practitioner is in a clinic or solo practice and other factors. Follow-up visits may range from $50 to $100.

The number of visits varies. A person with a more long-standing chronic illness, as, for example, chronic fatigue syndrome, may be seen every other month for two years, while someone with migraines may require only two or three total visits. According to Morrison, the more chronic or debilitated the organism, the longer it will take to cure them and they may need two or three different remedies over the course of their recovery process.

The remedies themselves are a negligible expense, usually around $5 to $15.

Most insurance companies reimburse for homeopathic physicians' services.

CHOOSING A PRACTITIONER

There is currently no national standard or certification for determining the competence of homeopaths, though this is the mission of the new Council for Homeopathic Certification (see page 163). Most practitioners are licensed primary care providers and the greatest number are M.D.s. However, other disciplines are also involved, including chiropractors, naturopaths, acupuncturists, nurses, nurse practitioners, physician's assistants, pharmacists, dentists, and veterinarians.

Any health care provider who does not consider him/herself a homeopath can still use homeopathic medicines. For example, there are certain remedies for injuries and for common pediatric problems such as teething, colic, or earache. There are no regulations on who can use homeopathic medicines.

Heath

A forty-four-year-old writer, Heath feared he was having symptoms of a heart attack: tightness or weight in his chest and extreme irregular heartbeats when he tried to exercise. He called his physician, a classical homeopath, who immediately ordered an electrocardiogram and blood work. The tests all came out normal. The physician determined the symptoms were stress related and prescribed a homeopathic remedy to be taken daily for five days. The symptoms began to diminish the first day and disappeared by the third. He felt an even higher level of energy and well-being after this episode.

In most states, the title "homeopath" is not legally protected. Connecticut, Arizona, and Nevada are the only states with such regulations and they have separate homeopathic medical boards.

There are a couple hundred lay homeopaths, i.e., unlicensed practitioners, the legality of whom is questionable. The issue hinges on whether the practice of homeopathy is considered the practice of medicine. Remedies are available over the counter and lay practitioners argue that they are not diagnosing or treating disease, but rather are doing something more along the lines of health consultation, akin to what a nutritional consultant might do.

Licensed practitioners, of course, argue that the practice of homeopathy is the practice of medicine. This controversy continues because the definition of practicing medicine varies from state to state.

Many lay practitioners are excellent practitioners simply because they have spent the time and effort necessary. The risk of working with a lay practitioner is the question of whether there is a serious medical condition that might go undetected and for which a more heroic type of medical treatment is needed. Some

161

people handle this concern by going to a physician to get thoroughly diagnosed and then going to a lay homeopath for treatment.

Of the range of degrees of preparation to practice homeopathy, classical homeopaths tend to be the most highly prepared, because a great deal of study is required to master the art of finding the constitutional remedy.

Training Programs

One way to assess the qualifications of a homeopath is to inquire about their training. The Council on Homeopathic Education has accredited five programs to date: National College of Naturopathic Medicine, Portland, Oregon; Bastyr University of Natural Health Sciences, Seattle, Washington; Ontario College of Naturopathic Medicine, Toronto, Ontario, Canada; Hahnemann Medical Clinic, Albany, California; and the International Foundation for Homeopathy, Seattle, Washington.

Other well-respected training programs include: Pacific Academy of Homeopathic Medicine, Berkeley, California (both laypeople and professionals), and New England School of Homeopathy, Amherst, Massachusetts. The National Center for Homeopathy, Alexandria, Virginia (page 164), offers summer courses for both laypeople and professionals, including dentists and veterinarians.

Since homeopathy is one of the most popular specializations in naturopathic medical schools, naturopathic homeopaths tend to have undergone more homeopathic training than M.D.s. Because M.D.s do not have such specialization available in medical school, they have to pursue it on their own and may not have had the number of hours of study in this discipline as their naturopathic counterparts. However, the training programs described above provide excellent training for M.D.s as well as other disciplines.

There are now available some correspondence courses that

provide surprisingly sound training that can augment any other training the person has (contact Homeopathic Educational Services, described on page 166, for information).

Certifying Organizations

While there is currently no universally accepted standard for the practice of homeopathy, there is growing demand for ways of identifying qualified homeopaths. The following organizations have taken steps in this direction, although it should be remembered that there are excellent practitioners who have not been certified.

The American Board of Homeotherapeutics offers the title "Diplomate in Homeopathy" (D.Ht.) to M.D.s, D.O.s, and D.D.S.s who pass a written and practical competency exam. A list of D.Ht.s is available from The American Institute of Homeopathy or The National Center for Homeopathy (see page 164).

Council for Homeopathic Certification was formed in 1992 by a coalition of several homeopathic associations to establish a national certification exam and code of ethics. It conducts a written and practical competency exam, leading to the designation "Certified in Classical Homeopathy" (C.C.H.) and listing in a national directory. Candidates for the exam must have had five hundred hours of training in homeopathy and one to two years experience. Address: P.O. Box 157, Corte Madera, CA 94976.

North American Society of Homeopaths (NASH) conducts a written and practical competency exam for nonphysician homeopaths, leading to the title "Registered-Society of Homeopathy, North America" or R.S.Hom. (N.A.). They publish a directory of R.S.Hom.s, a newsletter, educational materials, and a journal (*The American Homeopath*). NASH is currently involved in seeking state legislation for nonphysician homeopaths to receive health insurance reimbursement. Address: 10700 Old

County Rd. 15, #350, Minneapolis, MN 55441, phone (612) 593–9458.

Homeopathic Academy of Naturopathic Physicians offers the title "Diplomate in the Homeopathic Academy of Naturopathic Physicians" (D.H.A.N.P.), based on a written and practical competency exam. They publish *Similimum*, a quarterly journal on classical homeopathy, and a directory of diplomates. Address: P.O. Box 69565, Portland, OR 97201, phone (503) 795–0579.

Other Organizations

This tradition uses informal study groups as a vehicle for learning the theory and principles of homeopathy. Right now there are approximately two hundred such groups in the United States. According to Dana Ullman, president of Homeopathic Educational Services, contacting a local study group and asking who they recommend is probably the best way to find a practitioner. The National Center for Homeopathy maintains a listing of study groups.

The National Center for Homeopathy (NCH) is the largest organization, with approximately seven thousand members. Not all practitioners are members of NCH. It has a catalogue listing members by state, including a description of their training and whether they have been through a training program accredited by the Council on Homeopathic Education. They also publish a monthly magazine, *Homeopathy Today*. Address: 801 N. Fairfax St., #306, Alexandria, VA 22314, phone (703) 548–7790.

The American Institute of Homeopathy is the oldest national medical society of any kind in the United States and represents M.D.s, D.O.s, and D.D.S.s in the political and legislative arena. It is currently involved in seeking recognition of homeopathy as a medical subspecialty. It can provide a list of D.Ht.s certified by the American Board of Homeotherapeutics. Address: 1585 Glencoe, Denver, CO 80220, phone (303) 898–5477.

Rose

Rose, a four-year-old girl, developed a severe bladder infection after prolonged exposure to a hot tub. Her parents had raised her successfully on homeopathy so far and had managed to avoid antibiotics up to this time. As her temperature escalated they became increasingly alarmed. When it reached 105.4, she had a febrile convulsion. This was extremely frightening to them, and while cooling her down with moist sponges they rushed her to their family physician.

He told them such convulsions are common with such high fevers in children and it was not a life-threatening situation, but he advised antibiotics. They concurred and began what was to be a seven-day course of antibiotics. However, since the drugs require twenty-four hours to begin to take effect, the high fever continued.

For the next twenty-four hours, they were guided by a classical homeopath by phone in using homeopathy to control the fevers and prevent the convulsions. Each time Rose's fever would reach a point where she would begin to have symptoms signaling an impending seizure, they would pop the remedy into her mouth. Amazingly, her shaking would subside within three to five seconds and she would become calm. This happened several times through the night and into the next day until her temperature stabilized.

International Foundation for Homeopathy (IFH) is a non-profit educational foundation that trains both professionals and laypeople. The IFH has over 2500 members worldwide. They offer a 120-hour course for licensed professionals accredited by the Council on Homeopathic Education and have trained over

165

three hundred practitioners. They also publish a bi-monthly magazine, *Resonance*, and a directory of IFH-trained homeopaths. Address: 2366 Eastlake Ave. E, Suite 325, Seattle, WA 98102, phone (206) 304–8230.

Council on Homeopathic Education is the only accrediting organization for training programs in classical homeopathy. It sets minimum standards for number of hours and quality of instruction. Five programs have been accredited to date (see page 162). Address: 801 N. Fairfax, #306, Alexandria, VA 22314, phone (703) 548–7790.

Homeopathic Educational Services is a mail-order and retail company that provides books, tapes, remedies, and information about homeopathic resources worldwide. Its president is Dana Ullman, M.P.H., a homeopathic educator, activist, and author of *Discovering Homeopathy: Your Introduction to the Science and Art of Homeopathic Medicine* (Berkeley, CA: North Atlantic Books, 1991). Address: 2124 Kittredge St., Berkeley, CA 94704, phone (510) 649–0294.

Foundation for Homeopathic Education and Research is a nonprofit foundation that serves as a sponsor and clearinghouse for homeopathic research. Address: 2124 Kittredge St., Berkeley, CA 94704, phone (510) 649–8930.

Conclusion

Since homeopathy is a noninvasive and nontoxic approach, the choice of a practitioner need not necessarily be based on licensing or certification from the point of view of safety, except for ruling out serious health threats. Since there is no standard certification, your best bet in choosing a practitioner is to decide for yourself how important their training and credentials are for you and then give consideration to how comfortable you feel with them on a personal basis. You should certainly ask for references, from both professionals and former patients.

CHAPTER 6

MIND/BODY MEDICINE: THE DANCE OF SOMA AND PSYCHE

"The mind steadfastly refuses to behave locally, as contemporary scientific evidence is beginning to show. We now know, for example, that brainlike tissue is found throughout the body. . . . So, even from the conservative perspective of modern neurochemistry, it is difficult if not impossible to follow a strictly local view of the brain."

—LARRY DOSSEY, M.D.[1]

In the conduct of medical research, the existence of mind/body interactions has over the years been treated as a sort of hindrance. Such interactions are often lumped under the somewhat disparaging name of the placebo response. "Placebo" is a Latin term whose original meaning is "I shall please," and it refers to the mysterious and uncharted mechanisms by which the power of suggestion can result in a physiological change.

Ironically, the very scientific methods championed by mainstream medicine in the testing of drugs have provided the greatest scientific support for the existence and power of the mind/body connection. In fact, the mechanisms involved are so formidable that the standard research procedure requires separating out their effects from those of the drug.

Hence the power of mind/body mechanisms has been examined and measured in virtually thousands of drug studies. It is

in this sense that they have been verified and acknowledged by medical research to be a real and powerful phenomenon.

In the 1970s and 80s, researchers trained their sights more directly on these mechanisms. Herbert Benson, M.D., and his colleagues at Harvard Medical School led the way with the discovery of the relaxation response. This work has led to a cascade of findings about how mind/body mechanisms can be used for medically significant impact on hypertension, heart disease, cancer, and other conditions.

Today, leading edge programs for both patients and professionals are now conducted at Harvard's Mind/Body Medical Institute, New England Deaconess Hospital, Boston. And under Benson's direction, the institute is collaborating in the creation of other such programs at major medical centers around the nation.

In Benson's perspective, "We are part of mainstream medicine, we are not alternative. You might say that this was considered alternative years ago, but it is now mainstream."[2]

Taking Center Stage

Indeed he may be right. In early 1993, a widely reported study documented the surprising popularity of alternative medicine in this country. Published in *The New England Journal of Medicine* and led by Harvard researcher David Eisenberg, M.D., the study found that one in three adults had used some form of unconventional medicine. Of the varieties reported, mind/body techniques were the most frequently used.[3] The creation of the Office of Alternative Medicine at the National Institutes of Health followed a few months later. Shortly thereafter, mind/body medicine was brought into the living rooms of millions of Americans by a television series on PBS called *Healing and the Mind*, hosted by the popular journalist Bill Moyers.

The PBS series symbolized a highly visible milestone in the mainstreaming of what critics had previously considered a form of fringe medicine. Mind/body medicine (also known as behavioral medicine) is of course nothing new. The influence of the mind in healing is addressed in virtually every medical tradition, from the ancient teachings of Ayurveda to modern allopathy. What is new is the legitimization of research in this field to the point of government funding and the incorporation of mind/body programs into the offerings of major medical institutions, many of which are noted for their conservatism and scientific bent.

What is the emerging role of this work? Benson regards it as an integral part of comprehensive health care. He offers the metaphor of a three-legged stool: "One leg is pharmaceuticals, another is surgery, and the third is what you can do for yourself. Mind/body medicine is strengthening the third leg, integrated with the other two legs."[4]

KEY PRINCIPLES

The Biopsychosocial Perspective

In the late 1970s the eminent medical researcher George Engel of the University of Rochester made the bold statement that modern medicine needed a new way of thinking about health and illness.[5] He proposed what he called the biopsychosocial model, in which health is the outcome of many factors interacting together. This provides the theoretical framework underpinning mind/body medicine.

In this view, health is not just a matter of "the drugs keeping up with the bugs." Rather, health is determined by an interaction among our genetic vulnerabilities; environmental inputs such as germs, viruses, or pollutants; psychological factors such as stress, lifestyle, attitudes, and behavior; and social factors such as supportive relationships, economic well-being, access to health care, and family and community patterns of behavior.

169

Turning Down the Dial on Pain

Jim is a forty-six-year-old assembly line worker who received a disc injury in his neck and developed a chronic pain syndrome involving head, neck, arm, and shoulder pain. He was referred by his physiatrist to Karen Carroll, a biofeedback clinician practicing in Waterloo, Iowa, for pain control.

Carroll used EMG, first for general muscular tension and then for muscular tension around the upper body and neck. Jim was able to discover a direct connection between his thoughts, his level of nervous system arousal, muscular tension, and eventually his pain level.

After eight sessions spaced progressively further apart and accompanied by home practice of breathing exercises and progressive relaxation, his headaches and neck pain completely disappeared. He was then able to use physical therapy to further strengthen his neck and shoulders, and subsequently returned to work. He stated, "I never really knew what it felt like to relax until now." According to Carroll, this case illustrates the benefits of commitment to self-regulation and daily practice at home for someone who was motivated to avoid medication and surgery if possible.

Engel's perspective is gradually penetrating the thinking of mainstream medicine. When we look at the big picture of all the factors that influence health, we can see that many are within our direct control. Along with this new way of thinking has come a growing openness and receptivity to the contributions of mind/body approaches.

Mind/Body Communication

Our thoughts and feelings influence the body via two kinds of mechanisms: the nervous system and the circulatory system. These are the pathways of communication between the brain and the rest of the body.

The brain reaches into the body via the nervous system. This allows it to send nerve impulses into all the body's tissues and influence their behavior. The brain can thus affect the behavior of the immune system with its nerve endings extending into the bone marrow (the birthplace of all white cells), the thymus, the spleen, and the lymph nodes.

It also reaches into all the glands of the endocrine system, all the bones, muscles, all the internal organs, and even the walls of veins and arteries. It can influence the behavior of the heart with its nerves penetrating the heart tissue, affecting heart rate and other aspects of the heart's functioning. The entire body is literally "wired" by the brain.

The brain is also a gland. It manufactures thousands of different kinds of chemicals and releases them into the bloodstream. These chemicals circulate throughout the body and influence the activity and behavior of all the body's tissues. The brain could be described as the ultimate apothecary, producing many more drugs than science has ever invented.

The cells of the body have receptors on their surfaces that function somewhat like satellite dishes. These receptors receive the chemical messages being released by the brain and respond accordingly.

Finally, the mind/body connection is a two-way street. In addition to sending messages into the body's tissues, it also receives feedback, both in the form of nerve impulses and its own receptors that sense what chemicals are being released by other tissues in the body.

Research into how the brain can influence immune responses has given rise to the new field called psycho-neuro-immunology (PNI). Findings in this field have brought great hope to people dealing with such difficult illnesses as cancer, AIDS, CFIDS (chronic fatigue immune dysfunction syndrome), and other immune-related diseases.

It is only a matter of time before similar acronyms are defined for other fields such as psycho-neuro-cardiology (PNC), the study of the mind-heart connection, or psycho-neuro-hematology (PNH), the study of how the mind can influence blood-related disorders, such as clotting problems in hemophilia.

The Power of the Mind/Body Connection. One of the most stirring stories about the power of the mind/body connection concerns a man diagnosed with terminal cancer. Reported by Dr. Bruno Klopfer in the *Journal of Projective Techniques* in 1957, it involved a man with metastatic cancer and tumors that had spread throughout his body. The patient had tried every available form of medicine and his condition had hopelessly deteriorated to the point where he was bedridden and gasping for air. His doctors agreed that he had only a few days to live. Then the man heard about an experimental drug called Krebiozen, which was in the process of being tested. He insisted on being included in the experimental trials. His doctors, feeling he had nothing to lose and would soon be dead anyway, out of compassion agreed to give him the experimental drug. To their amazement, the man's tumors soon began to shrink dramatically and he was discharged from the hospital.

Two months later, the man read news accounts of the research on Krebiozen that reported serious doubts with the drug. Within a matter of days, the man's tumors had returned and were again threatening his life. His doctor cleverly convinced him that a new and more potent shipment had been received and proceeded to give him injections of plain water. His tumors once again began to shrink dramatically. He remained healthy for several more months until another news report declared "Nationwide AMA Tests Show Krebiozen to Be Worthless as a Cancer Treatment." The man died within two days.[6]

172

The Stress Response

The stress response is a set of changes in the body that result when the person experiences what they perceive to be a challenging or threatening situation. This matter of perceived threat is important because the effects of the stress response on the body are the same *whether the threat is real or just imagined in the mind.*

The magnitude of these changes is influenced by how serious the person thinks the situation is and what they think about their ability to handle the threat effectively (their appraisal of their ability to respond). Of course, the more confident the person is in their ability to handle a challenge easily, the less stress is involved. The more the person appraises the challenge as a threat—even at the subconscious level—the more intense will be the stress response.

Commonly called the fight-or-flight reaction, the stress response has the beneficial effect of preparing the body to function at a higher level of efficiency, which of course enhances the likelihood of survival. The physiological changes include:

- Increased blood pressure
- Increased respiratory rate
- Increased heart rate
- Increased oxygen consumption (burning of fuel)
- Increased blood flow to skeletal muscles
- Increased perspiration
- Increased muscle tone

While all these changes clearly contribute to one's ability to fight or flee in an emergency, they also have a downside. If the person is experiencing the stress response regularly and for extended periods of time, these physiological changes have the effect of weakening the body's resistance to illness and lowering the effectiveness of its mechanisms of self-repair.

The Relaxation Response

Another key principle is the relaxation response, which was discovered and named by Herbert Benson, M.D., and his colleagues in 1974.[7,8] They were studying a pattern of physiological changes that occurs in people practicing transcendental meditation (TM).

This pattern of changes has been found to represent a very beneficial state, one that is virtually a mirror image of the stress response. The relaxation response includes the following changes:

- Reduced blood pressure
- Reduced respiratory rate
- Reduced heart rate
- Reduced oxygen consumption (burning of fuel)
- Reduced blood flow to skeletal muscles
- Reduced perspiration
- Reduced muscle tension

The relaxation response is an antidote to the effects of the stress response and it has also been found to enhance the effectiveness of the body's defenses and self-repair mechanisms. Regular practice of techniques that elicit this response also brings improved emotional well-being and better handling of stressful life events.

The relaxation response is a physiological state, not a technique as such. As we shall see later, there are many techniques that can be used to produce it and, indeed, learning to do this is at the heart of mind/body medicine.

Coping, Emotions, and Health

Researchers have identified how the ways we cope with emotions and stressful situations—our coping styles—can influence

174

our physical health. Most firmly established are the links between coronary heart disease and the Type A behavior pattern. Type A is a way of coping characterized by constant hurriedness, intense competitiveness, and free-floating hostility.

A more recent concept is the Type C pattern, which in many ways is the polar opposite of Type A. It involves the nonexpression of anger and other unpleasant emotions such as fear and sadness, unassertive and overly appeasing behavior in relationships with others, and a preoccupation with meeting the needs of others, often to the point of extreme self-sacrifice. The theory of the Type C pattern was put forward by Lydia Temoshok, Ph.D., a leading health psychologist and PNI researcher. She has found compelling evidence for a link between emotional expressiveness and the progression of cancer.[9]

The middle ground, or Type B, is considered a more balanced way of coping that involves appropriate expression of all emotions and the ability to meet one's own needs while responding to those of others. People who cope in this more balanced way tend to be less at risk for serious illness. The cultivation of these behaviors is often a goal in mind/body medicine programs, especially for heart disease and cancer.

Lifestyle Change

The use of mind/body medicine takes place within a broader context of changing one's lifestyle to promote health. Making a daily practice of mind/body techniques is but one of several areas of lifestyle change that work together in a synergistic way. Other areas include proper diet, exercise, and social support.

While the health benefits of diet and exercise are obvious, there is a growing body of research now indicating that supportive interpersonal relationships are strongly associated with better health. They seem to ameliorate or buffer the harmful effects of stress on the body.

Turning Down the Pressure

Alice, suffering from chronic fatigue syndrome (CFS), undertook a two-week intensive treatment of intravenous Acyclovir therapy in the hospital. Acyclovir is a drug that inhibits the reproduction of herpes viruses, a family of viruses thought to be cofactors in CFS. One of the side effects of this therapy is elevated blood pressure, which needs to be closely monitored.

Alice was about halfway through her treatment protocol when she enrolled in a group mind/body medicine program. She brought her stainless steel drip apparatus with her from the hospital and stood it up beside her in the circle with the other patients and their spouses.

The first day involved a series of relaxation and deep breathing exercises. The next day Alice returned to the group bubbling with excitement. She reported that the previous evening her blood pressure had returned to normal. The nursing staff were mystified and wanted to know how she had done it.

VARIATIONS: THE MANY CONTEXTS OF MIND/ BODY MEDICINE

This field is uniquely cross-disciplinary, which accounts for its wide availability, helping make it the most commonly used form of alternative healing.

Its variety of techniques may be used by medical doctors, nurses, physician's assistants, naturopaths, osteopaths, practitioners of Chinese medicine and Ayurveda, bodyworkers, homeopaths, and chiropractors. Other human service providers such as psychologists, clinical social workers, marriage and family counselors, ministers, and hypnotherapists also use these tools. And of course there are very specialized applications for midwives, physical therapists, exercise physiologists, respiratory therapists, and others.

Mind/body approaches are generally taught either in office practice via private consultation with a health care provider or in group programs. Hospitals and other institutions offer various kinds of support groups or group therapy programs for people with cancer, heart disease, organ transplantation, and other conditions. Almost all such programs incorporate some use of mind/body techniques, such as relaxation exercises or imagery.

These methods are often taught to patients preparing to undergo surgery or other difficult treatments. Research has found such preparation to speed healing, reduce bleeding and complications, and result in earlier discharge from the hospital.

PROCEDURES AND TECHNIQUES

The repertoire of mind/body medicine includes all psychological strategies that directly influence physiological states. Following are the most commonly used methods.

Meditation

There are hundreds of varieties of meditation. The most basic approach for facilitating the relaxation response is that described by Herbert Benson. The process should take place in a quiet environment, a setting where one can be quiet, undisturbed, and in a comfortable position for at least fifteen to twenty minutes. Given this setting, there are only two essential steps: the silent repetition of a word, sound, phrase, or prayer and the passive return back to the repetition whenever other thoughts intrude.

Variations on these instructions are at the core of many forms of meditation from diverse spiritual traditions. The simplicity of these instructions, however, makes the approach available to virtually anyone, regardless of their spiritual or religious beliefs. This is because the person can use as their repetitive focus a prayer or any other words that reinforce their beliefs (e.g., "God is love"), thereby adding a further dimension of comfort to the experience.

Mindfulness

This is actually another approach to meditation, which involves the ability to focus completely on only one thing at a time. In other words, in mindfulness the mind is full of whatever is happening right now. This can include walking, cooking, sweeping the floor, dancing, watching a bird, hearing the sound of a river, or any other focus you may choose. Whenever thoughts intrude, you simply return your attention back to the focus. This is a traditional Buddhist approach and has been widely popularized by Jon Kabat-Zinn, Ph.D., in the Stress Reduction Clinic, University of Massachusetts Medical Center, Worcester.

Progressive Relaxation

This is another common approach to eliciting the relaxation response. In this technique the body itself is used as the focus of attention. It may be done either lying down or sitting. The technique involves progressing through the body one muscle group at a time, beginning with the feet, moving up the legs, and so on, spending approximately a minute in each area. For each muscle group, you hold or clench the muscles in the area for a count of ten and then release for a count of ten before moving on to the adjacent area.

The remaining techniques described below, while they also can lead to induction of the relaxation response, are also used for other purposes.

Mental Imagery

This involves using symbols to imagine that the changes you desire in your body are actually happening. For example, you might imagine that pain is melting away and dripping like a warm liquid out of your fingertips. Or you might develop an image of your immune cells actively subduing and preying on cancer cells or viruses, like birds of prey swooping down to engulf field mice in a meadow. This is a highly personalized technique and you would use images that are uniquely exciting and meaningful to you.

Studies of mental imagery have found that people can actually influence their immune functioning as well as significantly reduce pain and tension in the body with this method. But aside from the physiological benefits, which take some practice to achieve, there is also the knowledge that you are doing something to help yourself, channeling your energy into a healing activity. This in itself helps to improve emotional well-being and build a sense of self-efficacy or confidence, which research has found to improve immune functioning.

Autogenic Training

This approach involves using a combination of autosuggestion and imagery. Phrases are used to describe to oneself what changes in the body are desired as if they are happening now. For example, "My legs are warm and heavy," "All the muscles of my back are softening and melting," "I am calm," and "Warm, peaceful relaxation is flowing throughout my body." These phrases are repeated while maintaining one's focus on those parts of the body being addressed. Whenever the mind wanders, the attention is gently and passively returned to the focus.

Breath Therapy

A variety of breathing exercises can help one to release tension, anxiety, and pain. They can be used in conjunction with imagery or autosuggestion. They can also be used to encourage fuller breathing in general and give the body a greater supply of energy, which it can use for healing. It takes energy to fuel the body's self-repair mechanisms including the immune system. Since we take a thousand breaths every hour, each breath is an opportunity to contribute to a healing process.

Some breath therapy techniques use the breath in a calm, peaceful way to induce relaxation, to release pain, or to prepare for imagery. Another variety is Evocative Breath Therapy (EBT), which uses stronger breathing, sometimes accompanied by music, to stimulate emotions and emotional release.

Hypnosis

A simple description of hypnosis is offered by Karen Olness, M.D., of Case Western Reserve University who calls it "a form of self-induced, focused attention that can make it easier for you to relax or learn to control your body's functions."[10] It is this experience of extraordinary focus of attention that makes it possible to influence bodily states.

A Hike in the Tetons

Larry was a successful forty-two-year-old architect at the time he developed pancreatic cancer with metastases in 1978. He integrated meditation and imagery into his chemotherapy treatment and though the road was long, he recovered completely, with no further signs of cancer three years later.

He tells the following story about his devotion to doing his imagery practice:

"My girlfriend at the time and I had taken a back-packing trip to the Grand Tetons. This was nine months into my treatment. We'd get out there on the trail and after lunch, which was one of my times, I'd want to sit on the trail or on a rock, or lean against a tree and do my visualization.

"This woman was go-go-go, very achievement oriented. She was a very dynamic and pushy and controlling person. 'We're going to hike to this point, have lunch . . . by such and such a time we'll be at the campground,' and she would get terribly impatient with my after-lunch visualization.

"It started leading to more and more friction, but I maintained my ground. I was insistent that this is what I was going to do. By the time the trip was over, we weren't speaking. We flew back from Wyoming, not even sitting together on the plane, but that was very important for me, because I didn't often put myself first when it came to her."

Since his recovery, Larry has remained involved with a cancer self-help program as a lecturer in imagery. His story inspires many others to challenge difficult odds. There is no medical explanation for his recovery. The chemotherapy of the day was not considered curative for his condition, yet somehow he was able to marshall the resources to heal.

When in a hypnotic state, the mind is perfectly aware of the surroundings and the situation, but because it is so highly focused, it is able to concentrate on a task without being easily distracted. This enables the person to use imagery, relaxation, or autogenic suggestions in a richer, more powerful way.

Hypnosis is especially useful for relief from pain, reducing the distress from other symptoms or the side effects of treatment, and establishing a greater sense of control. Hypnotic states can be self-induced or facilitated by a hypnotist or hypnotherapist. Finally, it can help in overcoming one's resistance to healthful behavior change, such as reducing smoking or changing one's eating habits.

Biofeedback

Biofeedback uses special instruments attached to the body to give the person information about what is happening in the body. The instruments serve to amplify the signals that the person may not otherwise be able to detect so they can then use this visual or auditory feedback to learn to regulate certain bodily functions. Many people find this form of assistance very helpful for learning to relax.

The most commonly used form is *electromyographic* (EMG) biofeedback. An EMG sensor is attached to the skin and reveals the amount of electrical activity related to muscle tension in the area of the sensor. This is very useful in helping people learn to relax the muscles, for they have direct feedback—which may be visual readouts, lights, beeps, or tones—as to the degree of tension. This approach is often used for tension headaches and chronic pain conditions.

Other kinds of biofeedback include *thermal*, sensing the temperature of the skin as an indication of blood flow and relaxation; *electrodermal* (EDR), measuring subtle changes in amounts of perspiration; *finger pulse*, for measuring heart rate and force, useful for anxiety or cardiovascular symptoms; and monitoring *breathing patterns*—rate, volume, rhythm, and location (belly or chest) of each breath.

Biofeedback has many applications, such as headache and migraines, anxiety, chronic pain, teeth grinding and clenching, Raynaud's disease (vascular disorder causing cold hands and feet), incontinence, asthma, and muscle disorders (including helping people learn to reuse arms or legs that have been traumatized). Essentially any bodily process that can be measured can potentially be controlled or influenced through the help of these techniques.

SCIENTIFIC SUPPORT

There are four areas of research that support mind/body medicine: studies describing the physiology of mind/body interactions, those measuring the effects of mind/body therapy techniques, research on the health outcomes of structured mind/body programs employing a variety of techniques, and studies of cost effectiveness.

Mind/Body Interactions

The Mind/Heart Connection. Scientists have pieced together how stress affects the heart. This work is well summarized by Cynthia Medich, Ph.D., R.N., a cardiovascular specialist and researcher at the Mind/Body Medical Institute, Harvard Medical School and New England Deaconess Hospital, Boston. What Medich describes as the mind/heart connection involves the release of two kinds of stress hormones into the bloodstream: corticosteroids and catecholamines.

These hormones set off a cascade of changes in the body including increased platelet aggregation (tendency for blood

OAM-Funded Studies

Eight of the initial thirty studies funded by the Office of Alternative Medicine, National Institutes of Health, deal with mind/body medicine.

Biofeedback. Angele McGrady of the Medical College of Ohio in Toledo is studying the use of biofeedback-assisted relaxation in reducing the dosage of insulin required in type I insulin-dependent diabetes mellitus. The method is being studied as an alternative to increasing the dosage when the person is under stressful conditions. Richard Sherman at Fitzsimmons Army Medical Center in Aurora, Colorado, is evaluating biofeedback in treating chronic musculoskeletal low back pain and muscle-related orofacial pain.

Imagery. James Halper of Lenox Hill Hospital in New York City is conducting a controlled study of the benefits of guided imagery for patients with asthma.

Mary Jasnoski of George Washington University, Washington, D.C., is examining the effects of imagery on the immune system, with potential implications for use in cancer and AIDS.

Blair Justice of the University of Texas Health Sciences Center in Houston was funded to conduct a controlled study examining the effects of a group imagery/relaxation process on immune function and quality of life in breast cancer patients.

Hypnosis. Helen Crawford of Virginia Polytechnic Institute and State University in Blacksburg is examining how the use of hypnosis affects the electrophysiology of the brain in patients with low back pain. Carol Ginnandes of McLean Hospital in Belmont, Massachusetts, is studying whether hypnosis can be used to speed the healing of broken bones. Patricia Newton of the Good Samaritan Hospital and Medical Center in Portland, Oregon, is conducting a pilot study of the effects of hypnotic imagery on psychological and immunological factors in breast cancer patients.

clotting); increased coronary artery tone; a surge in coronary artery pressure; increased blood pressure, glucose levels, and lipid levels; a more rapid and powerful heartbeat; and, paradoxically, a constriction in the coronary arteries. In short, the demands on the heart all increase.[11]

With this understanding it is easy to see how individuals who experience stress on a chronic basis are at greater risk for heart diseases. This connection was dramatically illustrated in a study of air traffic controllers, considered to be in a very stressful occupation, who were found to have *five times* the incidence of hypertension as a comparison group of second-class airmen.[12]

Other research has been able to anticipate who will develop hypertension and heart disease. One study followed 1100 adults for twenty years. Those who had the highest levels of anxiety at the beginning of the study turned out to have the highest rates of hypertension two decades later.[13]

An eight-year study of over three thousand people found that those with the Type A behavior pattern were twice as likely as Type Bs to develop coronary heart disease.[14]

Depression has also been found to affect the heart adversely. A study of patients with a history of heart disease found that those who were also depressed were eight times as likely to develop ventricular tachycardia as the patients who were not depressed. (Ventricular tachycardia is a condition of abnormal and potentially deadly heart rhythms.)[15]

A ten-year study was conducted to follow the mortality rates of people who had experienced stroke. Those who had been diagnosed with either major or minor depression were 3.4 times as likely to have died within the follow-up period. The death rate among depressed patients with few social contacts was especially high: over 90 percent had died.[16]

In a study of 194 heart attack patients, those who reported lower amounts of emotional support in their lives were nearly three times as likely to die within six months as those with higher levels of emotional support.[17]

The Mind and Immunity. In addition to affecting the heart, the chemistry of the stress response has been found to lower immune functioning. This is illustrated by studies of the effects of exam stress on medical students that have found significant drops in the activity of natural killer (NK) cells[18] as well as in the numbers [19,20] of NK cells (NK cells are a key in fighting cancer cells and viruses) and a significantly lower percentage of T-helper cells in the blood[21,22] (the cells that arouse the immune response to fight off an infection).

In a study of recently divorced people, those who wanted the divorce, for whom it brought relief, were found to have better immunity than those who did not want the divorce.[23]

A study of the effects of stress on salivary immunoglobulin A (S-IgA, the antibody that fights infections in the mouth and throat) found that a higher frequency of daily hassles was significantly associated with lower levels of S-IgA. However, the effects were less severe in people who scored higher on a scale measuring sense of humor. This suggests that sense of humor can counter the negative effects of stress on the immune system.[24]

Research has shown that depression can have an adverse effect on immunity. A study that took place in a mental hospital compared natural killer (NK) cell activity in depressed patients, schizophrenic patients, and staff members. The patients with major depressive disorder had significantly lower NK functioning than schizophrenic patients and staff members.[25]

A study involved 132 college students to determine the effects of positive emotions on S-IgA levels. Half watched a morbid documentary about power struggles in World War II, while the other half watched an inspiring film about Mother Teresa, a Roman Catholic nun selflessly serving the poor and sick in Calcutta. The latter group had significantly increased S-IgA concentrations, indicating heightened immune responsiveness.[26]

Mind/body researcher Lydia Temoshok, Ph.D., studied the psychological factors associated with malignant melanoma. Among her findings was the discovery that emotional expressiveness was directly related to the thickness of the patients' tumors as well as the course of their disease.[27,28]

Major findings of Temoshok's research include the following:

- Patients who were more emotionally expressive had thinner tumors and more slowly dividing cancer cells.
- The more emotionally expressive patients had a much higher number of lymphocytes (immune cells) invading the base of the tumor.
- Patients who were less emotionally expressive had thicker tumors and more rapidly dividing cancer cells.
- Patients who were less expressive had relatively fewer lymphocytes invading the base of the tumor.

These findings helped contribute to the formation of the concept of Type C coping.

Can the immune system be trained to respond, like Pavlov's dog was trained to salivate at the sound of a bell? In a well-designed, controlled study, participants were given a sherbet sweet along with a subcutaneous injection of a chemical known to increase NK cell activity (epinephrine). After several administrations of this regime, the epinephrine was replaced by a useless saline injection. Remarkably, the participants still increased their NK cell activity in response to eating the sherbet accompanied only by the saline injection![29]

Techniques of Mind/Body Medicine

Some research on techniques has examined their effects on specific bodily functions such as immune responses, blood pressure, and heart rate. Other studies have looked at recovery from surgery, and still others have focused on psychological well-being and the quality of life.

Relaxation Training. This is by far the most widely studied subject in this tradition with hundreds of studies documenting its benefits. A few examples: Patients with ischemic heart disease who practiced the relaxation response daily for four weeks achieved significant reduction in the frequency of preventricular contractions.[30]

Patients with hypertension who took an eight-week (once a week) training program achieved significantly lower blood pressure and the benefits were maintained three years later.[31]

Patients receiving several kinds of elective surgery who were trained in relaxation had less surgical anxiety both before and after surgery. The intensity of their pain and their use of pain medication were both reduced.[32]

Also, a study of patients receiving angioplasty procedures showed significantly less anxiety, pain, and need for medication.[33] In patients receiving heart surgery, those who received the training had significantly lower incidence of postoperative supraventricular tachycardia.[34]

A controlled study of women with premenstrual syndrome (PMS) using the relaxation response twice daily for three months found a 58-percent reduction in the severity of their symptoms.[35]

Two studies found increased NK cell activity as a result of practicing the relaxation response. One, involving geriatric residents in nursing homes, also found indications of lower activity of herpes viruses. In addition, there were significant reductions in symptoms of emotional distress.[36]

Finally, in a study of exam stress in medical students, the more they practiced the relaxation response, the higher the percentage of T-helper cells circulating in their blood.[37]

Meditation. Of many various forms of meditation, TM has led the way in mind/body research. Over five hundred papers have been published in 108 scientific journals, authored by scientists at 211 research institutions and universities, in twenty-three countries worldwide. Studies of TM were instrumental in discovering the relaxation response and its benefits for hypertension. Other studies have found important benefits for such diverse populations as prison inmates, drug addicts, and Vietnam veterans suffering from posttraumatic stress disorders.

In one study, patients with hypertension who practiced TM twice daily for five to six months achieved significantly lower blood pressure.[38] In another, the effects of TM were compared to those of progressive muscle relaxation and usual care in hypertension. For those using TM, the decreases in systolic and diastolic blood pressure were twice as great as those for the subjects in the other groups.[39] As will be seen later, TM has also shown impressive effects in reducing the utilization rates of medical services.

Imagery. Imagery is often used in combination with relaxation and meditation. A controlled study of fifty-five women examined the effects of imagery and relaxation on breast milk production in mothers of infants in a neonatal intensive care unit. They received a twenty-minute audiotape of progressive relaxation followed by guided imagery of pleasant surroundings, milk flowing in the breasts, and the baby's warm skin against theirs. They produced more than twice as much milk as those receiving only routine care.[40]

In another study, a group of metastatic cancer patients using daily imagery for a year achieved significant improvements in NK cell activity and several other measures of immune functioning.[41]

At Michigan State University, researchers found that students could use guided imagery to improve the functioning of certain white cells called neutrophils, important immune cells in defense against bacterial and fungal infection. They could also decrease, but not increase, white cell counts. At one point in the study, a form of imagery intended to increase neutrophil count unexpectedly caused a drop instead. Subsequently, students were taught imagery explicitly intended to keep the neutrophil count steady, while increasing their effectiveness. Both of these goals were achieved.[42]

Breath Therapy. A study examined the effect of evocative breath therapy (EBT) on salivary immunoglobulin A (S-IgA). EBT involves abdominal breathing accompanied by music and posthypnotic suggestion to promote emotional arousal and release. Forty-five adults in a group therapy program for cancer showed

189

an average 46-percent increase in S-IgA levels after an hour-long EBT experience.[43]

Biofeedback. A controlled study of patients with irritable bowel syndrome found that biofeedback training brought a significant reduction in symptoms. This change was still present six months later.[44] Another controlled study found a 41-percent reduction in migraine headaches in patients using a thermal biofeedback procedure at home.[45]

Multistrategy Group Programs

Most organized mind/body therapy programs use a regimen of several techniques. Below are described some findings of such multistrategy programs for specific illnesses.

Hypertension. A group program for patients with hypertension included training in the relaxation response, nutrition, exercise, and stress management.[46] Findings included significant reductions in blood pressure, cholesterol, triglycerides, weight, body fat percentage, and psychological symptoms. Importantly, most of the benefits were intact when the patients were checked three to five years later.[47]

Surviving Heart Attacks. Patients recovering from myocardial infarction took a six-hour program of stress management training with mind/body techniques and emotional support. The result was a 50-percent reduction in subsequent rate of cardiac deaths.[48]

Reversing Heart Disease. A controlled study at the Preventive Medicine Research Institute, University of California, San Francisco, examined the effects of a multistrategy program on people with severe coronary heart disease. Patients were randomly assigned to either a usual care group or the experimental program.

The latter involved a regimen of dietary changes, exercise, yoga, and group support that included the practice of mind/body techniques. Those in the experimental program almost universally showed reductions in coronary artery blockage, while those with usual care generally showed more blockage.[49]

Benefits for Infertility. A ten-week group program for infertile women included training in the relaxation response with instructions for daily practice and training in stress management, exercise, nutrition, and group support. Results included decreases in anxiety, depression, and fatigue and increased vigor. Also, 34-percent of the women became pregnant within six months of the program.[50]

Reducing Symptoms of AIDS. In a controlled study, patients received group training in biofeedback, guided imagery, and hypnosis. Results included significant decreases in fever, fatigue, pain, headache, nausea, and insomnia. Vigor and hardiness also significantly increased.[51]

Another group program for HIV found significant improvement in emotional expression, sense of control over health, tension, anxiety, fatigue, depression, and total mood disturbance.[52]

Psychological Well-Being in Cancer. Fifty-nine patients took a ten-day, sixty-hour group program that includes imagery, relaxation training, lifestyle evaluation, emotional release therapies, group support, breath therapy, and exploring the personal meaning of illness. Results included significant improvements in emotional expressiveness, fighting spirit, quality of life, sense of control over health, and optimism—including patients with metastatic disease. These improvements were still present three months after completing the program.[53]

Psychological Well-Being and Immunity in Cancer. Sixty-six patients with malignant melanoma took a six-week structured group program that included health education, stress management, training in problem solving, and psychological support.

191

Josephine

Josephine, thirty-six, suffering from headaches, sought help from her physician. Her blood pressure was 150/100, she was twenty pounds overweight, and her cholesterol level was 280 mg/dl. She smoked a pack a day and did not exercise regularly. She was given a beta-blocker for high blood pressure, a cholesterol drug, and was told to lose weight and stop smoking.

Two months later her blood pressure was 160/102. She had lost no weight, she had not been able to stop smoking, and her cholesterol was 290 mg/dl. When asked why she hadn't cooperated with the recommendations she broke down in tears. She hadn't been able to afford the medications ($90/month). Her husband had left her and their two children after a stormy and abusive marriage, so she had been trying to work two jobs, felt depressed, was not sleeping well, and her headaches were now a daily occurrence.

She was referred to the Hypertension Clinic at the New England Deaconess Hospital, Boston, and participated in a twelve-week program of two-hour sessions with ten other participants. The program emphasizes the relaxation response, diet, exercise, and stress management. Her goals in the program were to control her blood pressure, lose weight, and stop smoking. During the program she regained some of her self-esteem, began to feel more hopeful, started sleeping better, was less irritable with her children, and was able to find assistance for child care and vocational training. She monitored her blood pressure once a day, which dropped to 124/90, and her medication was stopped. She was headache-free. She started walking daily and lost five pounds. Her cholesterol dropped to 220mg/dl. She practiced the relaxation response once a day and signed up for an assertiveness training class at the YWCA.

Before leaving the program, she outlined the situations that might be associated with relapse and developed a plan for action that included returning periodically for the drop-in groups for reinforcement. She also signed up for a SmokeEnders group to start after the program ended.[54]

Six months after the program, there were significantly lower levels of psychological distress and higher levels of positive coping methods in comparison to patients who did not have the program. There were also significant increases in the percentage of NK cells and in their functional effectiveness (cytotoxic activity).[55]

Increasing Survival Time in Malignant Melanoma. The patients who participated in the above study were followed for six years. A startling difference in death rates between the two groups was found. Of those who were in the control group (no group therapy), thirteen of thirty-four had a recurrence of cancer during the six years and ten died. For those who had the group program, only seven of thirty-four had recurrences and only three died.[56]

Increasing Survival Time in Breast Cancer. A ten-year controlled study was conducted with eighty-six women with metastatic breast cancer. Those who had a year of weekly group sessions had nearly double the survival time of those who did not have the group (averaging thirty-six months versus eighteen months). The group provided self-hypnosis and a form of therapy called "supportive-expressive therapy."[57]

Cost-Effectiveness

Aside from the medical and psychological benefits, one of the most important contributions of mind/body medicine is in reducing the costs of health care by reducing the utilization rates of expensive inpatient and outpatient services.

Dr. Elizabeth Devine of the University of Wisconsin School of Nursing in Milwaukee conducted an analysis of 191 different scientific studies in which surgery patients were taught simple mind/body techniques. She found an average reduction in the length of hospital stay of 1.5 days (12 percent). This of course translates into enormous savings, considering the cost of a day of hospitalization. Results also included faster recovery from surgery, fewer complications, and reduced postsurgical pain.[58]

Other studies have found reduced utilization rates for outpatient medical services. For example, in one study 109 chronic pain patients took a ten-session outpatient group mind/body program. A 36-percent reduction in total monthly clinic visits for pain management was found in the first year after the program.[59]

Another study looked at the medical care utilization rates of two thousand regular practitioners of TM, comparing them with 600,000 other members of the same insurance carrier. For children and young adults the reduction for inpatient services was 50 percent and for older adults it was 69 percent. The reductions for outpatient services were 47 percent for children, 55 percent for young adults, and 74 percent for older adults.

The same pool of TM practitioners were compared to five other health insurance pools, showing 55 percent fewer visits for benign or malignant tumors, 87 percent fewer visits for heart disease, 30 percent fewer visits for infectious diseases, 31 percent fewer visits for mental disorders, and 87 percent fewer visits for diseases of the nervous system.[60]

STRENGTHS AND LIMITATIONS

The greatest strengths of mind/body medicine are in stress-related conditions and chronic illnesses. It also has a great deal to offer in terms of relief of the symptoms of acute illnesses as well as relief from the side effects of treatment such as surgery, radiation, or chemotherapy in cancer.

This is obviously a complementary form of medicine rather than a primary treatment for major diseases. However, while it is usually thought of as supportive rather than curative, there are illnesses that do not respond to conventional medical treatment and for which mind/body medicine offers a way of gaining some relief and promoting recovery.

One point of controversy that often arises in this tradition is the question of whether its use implies an assumption that one's illness must have been caused by the mind in the first place. For example, there are those who question whether this approach should be applied to cancer because to use it might suggest that the person brought the cancer upon themselves. This is an unnecessary assumption since the mind/body connection can be exploited regardless of the cause of an illness.

The leading PNI researcher Alastair Cunningham, who holds Ph.D.s in both psychology and immunology, articulates this point well: "Although epidemiological considerations suggest that the contribution of psychological factors to cancer onset is small . . . no upper limit to what can be achieved by psychotherapy is necessarily thereby set: the relative influence of the psyche on outcome may be greatly expanded by such therapy, overriding the usual progression of disease."[61]

One limitation is that the methods require an ability to sit quietly and in some cases focus the mind on a technique. Some people suffering from extreme symptoms of disease may at times have difficulty following through with a routine of regular practice. Those who do best are able to sustain a regular practice and achieve cumulative benefits over time.

It should also be remembered that while there have been many studies documenting significant effects of mind/body techniques,

A Walk on the Beach

Heidi, thirty-five, was scheduled for a round of chemotherapy for breast cancer. The treatment was to take place on Friday and she and her husband had tickets to fly to Hawaii on Saturday for a week's vacation.

As is routine, she was called into the treatment center for a blood check on the Monday before to make sure her white cell count had recovered enough from the previous treatment to allow her to qualify for the next one. To her shock, she was told that her white count was only about half what it should be and she would probably have to forego her vacation.

For four days she practiced imagery intensively several times a day, concentrating on raising her white count. She used images of the bone marrow releasing a steady, strong flow of white cells into her bloodstream and spreading throughout her body. She also imagined directing her breath into the bone marrow and thereby nourishing the stem cells (that produce the white cells) so that they could grow and release more white cells.

On that Friday, she went in for another blood test. Her white count had more than doubled. She was able to have the treatment and the next day was able to walk on the beach with her husband.

there are different kinds of significance. Statistical significance means that there is a measurable effect happening, but this does not guarantee that the effect is strong enough to cause tangible medical benefits.

Clinical significance, on the other hand, means that actual medical benefits have indeed been observed. The studies reporting a major change in the overall course of an illness or even longer survival time in cancer provide the best examples of clinically significant findings.

Hence a person may use mind/body techniques religiously and practice them perfectly with real commitment and still not get the medical benefits they desire. The degree of the contribution will vary from one person to the next, depending in part on the severity of the illness.

When people do not understand these limitations and have unrealistic expectations, they are at risk of feelings of failure, self-blame, depression, or disappointment that may arise when such expected results are not forthcoming. This is called the *psychosocial morbidity* of mind/body medicine. Patients and practitioners alike must endeavor to keep a realistic perspective on mind/body medicine, not overrating but also not underrating it.

THE PRACTITIONER-PATIENT RELATIONSHIP

Mind/body techniques are often used in the context of psychotherapy or group therapy. These situations offer the opportunity for addressing other important aspects of coping with an illness. Often it is important to deal with the emotional aspects of an illness before one can comfortably or confidently pursue use of the mind/body techniques.

In this sense, this is a relatively practitioner-dependent tradition. However, the professional is not so much a healer as a teacher. Once the methods are learned, you can use them on your own at home in the form of a daily practice. And of course there are other ways of learning the techniques such as books and tapes. Some highly motivated people are able to develop a fruitful practice without professional guidance, but such guidance is still advised, especially in using such methods with a more serious illness.

The Vital Fluid

Carol Anne was scheduled to undergo a complicated abdominal surgery to remove a cancerous tumor. Her surgeon told her that patients undergoing this procedure typically lose ten to eleven units of blood.

For several days prior to the surgery, Carol Anne practiced a form of imagery in which she pictured her body going through the surgery without losing any blood, the tissues knitting back together smoothly, no complications, and a speedy recovery. She also imagined the look on the surgeon's face when he realized that no blood had been lost.

The day after the surgery, the surgeon came into her room and congratulated her on how well she had come through the ordeal. To his amazement, she had required only one unit of blood. When she told him of her preparations, he smiled and walked out shaking his head.

EVALUATING PERSONAL RESULTS

The results of mind/body techniques may be immediately apparent with changes in mood, pain, or physiological state. This is one of the things that is appealing about this tradition. The body gives direct feedback as to the impact of the technique. In fact, the subjective experience is the most important way of evaluating results.

This is consistent with the advice of Carl Simonton, M.D., who first popularized the use of imagery with cancer. According to Simonton, the criterion of successful imagery practice is whether the person feels hopeful, powerful, and optimistic after doing it. This is much more important than the details of the images or whether they followed someone else's particular guidelines.[62] Research has also confirmed that feeling confident in one's ability to influence his or her health will in itself reduce the degree of stress they feel and have its own health-promoting effects.

Beyond the patient's subjective impressions, other means of evaluating results are biofeedback equipment or lab test results.

RELATIONSHIP TO OTHER FORMS OF MEDICINE

Mind/body medicine is usually used in the role of complementary therapy. This means it works alongside other treatment in a supportive way. I like this term because it communicates a cooperative partnership rather than being exclusive of other traditions. In fact, all medical traditions now include within them some attention to mind/body interactions and ways of working with them.

COSTS

The economics of mind/body medicine are another source of its appeal. Other than for the individual consultations or training programs one might engage to use this approach, there are no inherent costs in using this tradition. Many hospitals or community agencies offer group support programs free of charge that teach the techniques. There are also nonprofit organizations such as the Centers for Attitudinal Healing and the Wellness Community, both with nationwide chapters, who offer free group programs that include mind/body techniques.

Beyond the free or low-fee services mentioned above, services provided by professionals are often covered by health insurance if offered by a licensed primary care provider or a licensed mental health professional (psychologist, clinical social worker, marriage and family counselor). Coverage by the latter disciplines would usually be under the category of individual or group psychotherapy. Typical fees range from $40 to $100 or more for individual sessions and $25 to $50 for group sessions.

There are also many audiotape programs for home use that can be surprisingly effective and inexpensive.

CHOOSING A PRACTITIONER

Mind/body medicine knows no disciplinary bounds. There are no standardized credentials or requirements to use in evaluating one's preparation in these approaches. Because most techniques are not very complicated anyway, what is probably more important is that the practitioner is competent in having a therapeutic relationship and also has a healthy regard for the limitations and appropriate uses of mind/body techniques.

The techniques themselves are usually quite familiar to anyone who is trained in the mental health disciplines and other health care providers who received mental health training. Many training programs in the mental health disciplines include courses and experience in the field of behavioral medicine. Of course, licensing by the state is usually a good place to start for any such provider.

Beyond general licensing, there are numerous organizations and training programs in mind/body techniques that offer their own advanced certification. Such certification is by no means necessary in order for a person to be competent in a technique, although it can lead to a higher degree of skill and competence in specific techniques.

Most but not all such programs of advanced certification require the practitioner to be licensed in a professional discipline. A noteworthy exception in this regard is hypnotherapy, which in many states is acknowledged as a distinct profession without being linked to a specific academic discipline. Some states limit the practice of hypnosis or hypnotherapy to licensed therapists. Others allow it to be practiced by lay hypnotists but limit the scope of problems that can be addressed.

Organizations and Resources

The Mind/Body Medical Institute, Division of Behavioral Medicine, New England Deaconess Hospital offers group mind/body programs for different illnesses. They also have affiliate programs nationwide and conduct clinical training several times each year under the direction of Herbert Benson, M.D., and faculty. Address: 1 Deaconess Rd., Boston, MA 02215, phone (617) 632–9525, FAX (617) 632–7383.

The Cancer Support and Education Center conducts retreats and group programs for people with cancer and other serious illnesses. The program includes in-depth work with the emotional aspects of illness, as well as imagery, movement, deep relaxation, breath therapy, and nutrition. Address: 1035 Pine St., Menlo Park, CA 94025, phone (415) 327–6166, FAX (415) 327–2018.

Commonweal Cancer Help Program conducts a week-long retreat several times each year for cancer patients. The program focuses on informed choice among both conventional and alternative cancer treatments, and also includes mind/body and other holistic therapies. Address: P.O. Box 316, Bolinas, CA 94924, phone (415) 868–0970.

Stress Reduction Clinic, University of Massachusetts Medical Center, directed by Jon Kabat-Zinn, Ph.D., conducts an eight-week program and a five-day residential program in mindfulness training and stress reduction. Address: UMMC, Worcester, MA 01655, phone (508) 856–1616.

Insight Meditation Society and *Insight Meditation West* offer workshops and retreats nationwide in mindfulness meditation, also called vipassana meditation. Address: IMS, Pleasant St., Barre, MA 01005, phone (508) 355–4378; IMW, P.O. Box 909, Woodacre, CA 94973, phone (415) 488–0164.

201

The Long-Lost Brother

A meditation teacher and mystic living in northern California came from a family with the hereditary condition of polycystic kidney disease. At age forty-four he began to have the typical symptoms of breakdown in kidney function and by age sixty-three he was on the waiting list to receive a kidney transplant.

He was expecting a two-year wait and had already been using kidney dialysis for ten months. However, a longtime student and devoted friend heard of his need and immediately volunteered to donate a kidney to him.

Having taught for many years how to understand and communicate with the subconscious, he developed his own plan to prepare his body to receive the foreign organ and accept it easily without being rejected by his immune system. He used meditation, inner dialogues with his subconscious, hypnosis, and affirmations to help his body "welcome the kidney like a long-lost brother." His quick recovery and the rapid rate at which his antirejection medication was able to be reduced afterward led his physicians to regard him as a model case.

According to John Soos, Ph.D., a clinical psychologist working with organ transplantations in Vancouver, Canada, mind/body medicine can indeed "instruct the immune system to *improve* its functioning against germs while at the same time recognizing and tolerating the transplanted organ as an integral part of the new body image."[63,64]

The Center for Mind/Body Medicine has both residential and outpatient programs. Developed under the guidance of Deepak

Chopra, M.D., it also provides education and training programs in Ayurveda for laypeople and health care providers. Address: P.O. Box 1048, La Jolla, CA 92038, phone (619) 794–2425, FAX (619) 794-2440.

Maharishi Ayur-Ved Products International provides referrals to local resources for training in transcendental meditation (TM). Address: P.O. Box 49667, Colorado Springs, CO 80949–9667, phone (800) 255–8332.

The Academy for Guided Imagery provides training for professionals in the use of guided imagery. Address: P.O. Box 2070, Mill Valley, CA 94942, phone (800) 726–2070 or (415) 389–9324, FAX (415) 389–9342.

Biofeedback Certification Institute of America provides a directory of certified biofeedback practitioners, including their background and experience. Address: 10200 W. 44th Ave., Suite 304, Wheatridge, CO 80033, phone (303) 420–2902.

American Chronic Pain Association manages a list of over five hundred support groups internationally, and publishes workbooks and a newsletter. Address: P.O. Box 850, Rocklin, CA 95677, phone (916) 632–0922.

American Society of Clinical Hypnosis (ASCH) is the largest and most highly accredited organization for hypnotherapists. The ASCH sponsors the American Board of Clinical Hypnosis, which certifies practitioners, and maintains a referral list of professionally trained and licensed hypnotherapists. Address: 2200 East Devon Ave., Suite 291, Des Plaines, IL 60018, phone (708) 297–3317, FAX (708) 297–7309.

American Council of Hypnotist Examiners (ACHE) provides a referral list of professionally trained hypnotists and hypnotherapists certified by ACHE. It does not require licensure in a health or mental health profession. Address: 312 Riverdale Dr., Glendale, CA 91204, phone (818) 242–5378.

Center for Attitudinal Healing has support groups throughout the nation for people with chronic or life threatening illness. Address: 33 Buchanan, Sausalito, CA 94965, phone (415) 331–6161.

Wellness Community has chapters throughout the nation that conduct support groups for people with chronic or life threatening illness. Address: 2716 Ocean Park Blvd., Suite 1040, Santa Monica, CA 90405, phone (310) 314–2555.

Audiotape programs applying methods of mind/body medicine are available from many individual practitioners throughout the country. See About the Author in the back of this book for one resource.

Conclusion

Above all, mind/body medicine is an approach that requires your own participation. It does not require working with a practitioner, but if you choose to, it is important that you work with someone with whom you have a good rapport and whose style and manner you find comfortable. Often the practitioner's voice alone is enough to either draw or repel some people.

Beyond the issues of appropriate licensing or certification, it is important that the practitioner have a balanced perspective of both the limits and possibilities of mind/body medicine. Anyone who promises a cure of a serious illness is immediately suspect. The wisest practitioners take a conservative approach in extolling the virtues of this tradition.

Finally, structured group programs have a lot of advantages over individual treatment. If you can find a group program, you can gain a great deal of reinforcement for healthful behavior change from the mutual support of others who share the healing journey with you.

CHAPTER 7

OSTEOPATHIC MEDICINE: STRUCTURE AND FUNCTION AS ONE

"There is no real difference between structure and function: they are two sides of the same coin. If structure does not tell us anything about function, it means we have not looked at it correctly."
— ANDREW TAYLOR STILL[1]

Osteopathic medicine was founded by the American physician Andrew Taylor Still (1828–1917). A surgeon during the Civil War, Still lived during an era when medical education was not organized and most medical schools were private proprietary businesses, often with just a few faculty. Also there were only a limited number of allopathic techniques available, and surgical methods had not been developed to a very high degree.

An historic account published in 1918 by osteopathic professor Michael Lane, Ph.D., D.O., states that in Still's day "there was in America scarcely a handful of physicians of high scientific type. There were no discoveries made in America, and such medicine as was here was of the distinctly old style, crude and backward, and loaded with many of the superstitious beliefs and practices that had marked the medicine of Europe before the days of Schwann and Pasteur . . . and of other pure scientists whose work did so much to place medicine on a pedestal higher than that of mere experience and empiricism."[2]

Still was both a practitioner and researcher. Motivated in part by the deaths of his wife and children from spinal meningitis and his resulting disaffection with the conventional medicine available, in 1872 he formulated a theory of what today we might call holistic medicine. Osteopathic theory emphasizes the integration of the body's communication and regulatory mechanisms, the inherent defenses and healing powers of the body, the special role of the musculoskeletal system in relation to the organ systems, and an emphasis on health promotion as well as combating disease.[3]

Still formed the first school of osteopathic medicine in 1892. It was a four-year medical school with the basic core curriculum of allopathic schools of his day, augmented by his osteopathic theory and manipulation techniques.

He was fascinated by the relationship between structure and function. To him the musculoskeletal system played a much more key role in health than that attributed to it by his allopathic contemporaries. He observed that joint mechanics, the action of muscles, ligaments, joint surfaces, and joint motion all influenced the vascular (blood) and nervous systems.

The vascular and nervous systems were thought of as the main communication and regulatory mechanisms of the body, responsible for the health of all its organs and tissues. By using a variety of manipulative therapies, the blood supply and nerve supply throughout the body could be enhanced, thus allowing the body's inherent forces to maintain and assist in the restoration of health.[4] This emphasis on the manipulation of the musculoskeletal system is what gave rise to the name "osteopathy," in which *osteo* refers to the skeletal system and *pathy* means dysfunction.

The general osteopathic theory also held that "lesions," or disturbances of particular regions of the spinal column, caused disease ("somatic dysfunction") in the organs that are fed by the nerve impulses coming from those areas. To Still and his followers, this relationship between structure and function was considered the key in the development of most disease. This focus was quite different from that of the allopathy of the era, which was not concerned so much with causation of disease but rather with surgery and pharmacological advances for the control of symptoms.

The two camps diverged further as allopathy became much more highly organized politically and economically. Osteopathic medical schools and hospitals evolved separately from those of allopathy. Though they taught and practiced the full range of medicine and surgery, osteopathic physicians were not accepted by allopathy and were not allowed to practice in allopathic hospitals. In fact, until the 1940s, they were denounced by the AMA as cultists.

The allopathic medical degree took the lead in being institutionalized as the credential required for licensure for physicians in many states. Nevertheless, osteopathic physicians made gradual progress toward acceptance as their academic curriculum and training programs became recognized as equivalent to those of allopathy. By 1972, all fifty states had accepted D.O.s as qualifying for state licenses as physicians. It was, however, many more years before they were able to gain full access to many hospitals.

Current Status

Today there are about fifty thousand D.O.s in this country as compared to over 600,000 M.D.s. Osteopathic physicians are eligible for full membership in the AMA though they also maintain their own organization, the American Osteopathic Association (AOA). Many allopaths have sought training in osteopathic manipulation both to augment their practice and as a means toward helping them gain residencies in traditionally osteopathic settings. Such training for M.D.s is now accredited through the American Academy of Family Practice.

The relationship between the two traditions remains an interesting one. Osteopathic physicians view themselves as a "sepa-

Mary

Mary, twenty-eight, had been suffering from mitral valve prolapse for five years. Symptoms included anxiety, a sinking sensation in the chest with premature heartbeats, episodes of tachycardia, and fluttery feelings in the chest when the heart jumps out of rhythm. She had been taking Inderal, the common drug for this condition, a beta-blocker that blocks the effects of adrenaline on the heart.

Her osteopathic physician observed that she had a long thorax and a short left leg. With the left-twisting mechanism in her pelvis, her lumbar spine bent to the right and her chest bent to the left. Her head ended up leaning a little bit to the left and as she would walk her spine would favor the left-twisting motion. Her spine was twisted in such a way that the pressure was greatest on the third thoracic vertebra (T3).

Over a series of five sessions her spine was manipulated and she was given a progressively higher heel lift to wear in the left shoe. Her symptoms disappeared and she took herself off Inderal after two treatments.

As Carlisle Holland, D.O., explains, "If you develop a rotated segment in T2 or T3, that affects the atrium of the heart, and very often a patient will have preventricular contractions, mitral valve prolapse symptoms, and palpitations. The rotated segment causes 'facilitation,' which means the neurons fire more than normally and the heart becomes stimulated more easily.

"I put her in a heel lift, leveled her pelvis, mobilized her upper chest, and taught her how to stretch her upper body and maintain her posture, and she quit having mitral valve prolapse symptoms. Inderal suppresses the symptoms by interrupting the twisted segment's effect on the heart. You're treating a somatic dysfunction with a drug, but you're not getting to the cause."

rate but equal" profession. According to William Anderson, D.O., past president of the AOA, "We want to be treated as equally qualified physicians and have the same practice rights, but that does not mean abandoning the osteopathic profession to join the AMA. We believe the public interest is best served by having the two organizations. The AMA has historically had a monopoly on medicine in the United States, and monopoly is not good in any field. . . . Osteopathic physicians in many cases have made allopathic medicine better, have made allopathic physicians practice better."[5]

Anderson points out that there are some differences in the missions of the two professions. "We bring a history of being the premier providers of primary care, especially in underserved areas. While we are only 5 percent of the physician population, we represent as many as 15 percent of physicians who practice in communities of under ten thousand people."

He elaborates on this theme of service in the underserved and rural areas: "There is a niche in health care in America that is being filled by osteopathic physicians, and we want to continue to fill that niche. It is consistent with health care reform that we have more primary care physicians that are willing to go into the underserved areas." With about half its practitioners in primary care, Anderson sees the tradition as uniquely in step with the health care reform movement.

Education

Today there are seventeen osteopathic medical schools, for which the AOA is the approving body. The AOA in turn is accredited by the U.S. Department of Education for this purpose. There are also about two hundred AOA-approved teaching hospitals.

The curriculum is identical to that of allopathic medical schools with two exceptions. One is a greater emphasis on preventive medicine. The second is the addition of specialized training in treatment of the musculoskeletal system and manipulative therapies.

Given the fact that osteopathic medicine incorporates allopathic training, the interesting question arises as to whether this should be considered a form of alternative medicine. When asked this question, Anderson states very firmly, "We are not alternative. We are mainstream." To the layperson, of course, it represents an alternative to conventional allopathy by virtue of its use of manipulative therapies.

KEY PRINCIPLES

Holism

The term "holistic," which has come into vogue only in the last thirty years, refers to a perspective in which the body's systems are considered to be interdependent parts of a greater whole. This was a core principle of traditional osteopathic theory in that an integrated or balanced musculoskeletal structure was held to be reflected in optimal physiological functioning. The osteopathic view also includes psychological and emotional influences, as well as those systems outside the person—the familial and societal—as playing a role in the individual's health.

Structure and Function

Structure and function are interrelated and no condition exists in the human body where one does not affect the other.

Restrictions in structure lead to problems in function and problems in function will produce palpable structural changes. Anderson notes that the psyche and emotional life of the person are affected by the musculoskeletal structure and vice versa: "Ulcers, hypertension, and many other disease entities are not purely physiologic manifestations. They can also be reflective of emotional and structural abnormalities."

It follows that manipulation of structure affects function. Anderson offers the following illustration: "In hypertension, the cardiovascular system is seen as regulated by the sympathetic nervous system through the spinal segments with the ganglia that parallel the spinal cord. If there is a malalignment in the vertebral spinal segment, this can affect the function of the sympathetic ganglia and can in turn affect blood pressure.

"Hence, in treating hypertension, we can't just use medication. We have to look at the impact that the malalignment affecting the sympathetic ganglia would have on the cardiovascular system. We would use conventional allopathic drugs along with manipulation, since it has been demonstrated repeatedly in clinical studies that blood pressure can be effectively lowered by manipulation."

"The Rule of the Artery Is Supreme"

Any condition of illness is responsive to improvement in blood circulation, which is responsible for introducing essential nutrients to, and releasing toxins from, all the tissues of the body. Still was the first to make this observation and incorporate it into his philosophy. Hence the effects of structural manipulation on blood circulation are an important part of osteopathic theory.

Homeostasis

The body has an innate tendency toward health or homeostasis. When the body is injured or traumatized by illness, its initial

Sister Anne

A thirty-three-year-old nun and schoolteacher had been suffering from rheumatoid arthritis for fifteen years. Her treatment had included a six-month stay in an arthritis hospital as well as the conventional injections and other medications. She had been using a wheelchair, crutches, and a cane.

She was told by her physicians, "You're not going to die *from* this disease, you'll die *with* it. It's going to be bad if you walk around a lot. Use the wheelchair." She was also informed that she might need a hip replacement, which she found frightening.

Upon deciding to do some volunteer work at a free clinic in Clearwater, Florida, she met John Upledger, D.O. Upledger told her he could make her pain-free, but she was skeptical because of all the treatment she had been through.

Over a period of eighteen months he treated her with general osteopathic manipulation, acupuncture, CranioSacral Therapy,™ and manipulation under anesthesia and her condition gradually improved. Today, twenty years later, she still functions without gold shots, crutches, or a wheelchair. "I still have some bad days," she states, "but they're nothing like before."

Her involvement with osteopathic medicine did not stop with her own treatment. At Upledger's encouragement, she applied to Michigan State University College of Osteopathic Medicine and was accepted. Today Sister Anne Brooks, D.O., operates the Tutwiler Clinic as one of only three physicians in Tallahatchie County, Mississippi.

"It's not just that osteopathic medicine made me better that made me want to become a physician. The encouragement of John that I could do what to me was impossible—not only regaining control over my health, but also going back to school—taught me a lesson about hope. I try to give that to my patients."

One of the more special cases in her career illustrates the versatility of some osteopathic physicians.

"I had a priest who was unable to raise his arms when he celebrated mass because of arthritis pain. I used acupuncture on him and he recovered the mobility of his hands and arms. He was treated weekly for three to four months."

response is to attempt to restore homeostasis. However, there is a limited amount of vitality that it has to handle the problem. If it is unable to resolve the problem completely, the problem may move from an acute to a chronic state. In effect, the body decides "this is the best that I can do" and still seeks to maintain homeostasis, albeit at a lower level of functioning than would be optimal.

Osteopathic medicine would define health as being the optimal state of balance or homeostasis among the body's systems.

Restimulation

The human body is believed to have the innate ability to heal itself. Treatment is intended to restimulate the body to more effectively use this innate ability. Through hands-on manipulative techniques, medication, exercise, or appropriate behavior change, the body is stimulated to reach a higher degree of homeostasis. In other words, treatment helps the body move further toward reintegration than it may have otherwise been able to.

Chronic problems arise when the body does not have enough vitality to handle the problem on its own. It may then encase the trauma, in a sense trying to ignore it. The person may develop holding patterns in areas of the body where there is no motion or decreased motion. Through treatment the practitioner is helping the body "remember" and return to a state of health that it cannot re-create on its own.

Somatic Dysfunction

Osteopathic theory holds that there is a state in tissue called somatic dysfunction that precedes the development of disease. This is a state in which the tissue is no longer working as it should, but actual distortion in shape or histological change at the cellular level has not yet occurred.

According to Carlisle Holland, D.O., of Santa Rosa, California, "The important thing about believing that there is a stage that *precedes* disease is we also believe that it is reversible. If you know how to restore proper texture and motion, you can take a person out of that state of dysfunction. This is the key concept that is missing in allopathy."

Preventive Focus

A strong emphasis in osteopathic medicine is lifestyle education, including nutrition and exercise. Osteopathic medical school curricula have specific courses in nutrition and lifestyle and the profession has a specialty in preventive medicine.

VARIATIONS WITHIN THE TRADITION

With regard to what is historically unique about osteopathic medicine—the use of osteopathic manipulation—there are two broad varieties of practitioners. The first group are those who consider manipulation as the centerpiece of their practice and do not wish to be characterized as conventional physicians equivalent to allopaths, even though they are licensed as such.

The second group, the majority, liberally use allopathic approaches in their practice and align themselves politically and professionally with allopathy, although some augment their practice with osteopathic manipulation. To many of these, osteopathic medical education was mainly a vehicle for becoming a licensed physician and the unique heritage of the tradition is not emphasized so much in their practice.

It is estimated that about half to two-thirds of osteopathic physicians use manipulation fairly regularly and about 5 to 10 percent specialize in it.

Specializations

Osteopathic physicians are able to practice in all the specialties in which allopaths do. There are over seventy board specialties that are practiced by D.O.s. However, because this is a tradition with a strong emphasis on preventive and holistic medicine, about half the graduates of osteopathic medical schools go into primary care. This compares with about 12 percent of M.D.s going into primary care and 88 percent into other specialties. Recently the AOA has developed the Primary Medical Initiative, a six-year medical school program that graduates fully qualified primary care physicians.

Integrative Medicine

In a sense osteopathic medicine is inherently an integrative form of medicine since it combines allopathic approaches and more holistically oriented, manipulative approaches.

215

Like their allopathic counterparts, osteopathic physicians are free to integrate modalities from such diverse traditions as homeopathy, naturopathy, Chinese medicine (medical acupuncture is taught in some schools), Ayurveda, mind/body medicine, and bodywork. Many create their own personal synthesis of approaches and a few even devote their practice exclusively to one of these other traditions. (The concept of integrative medicine is discussed further in Chapter 10.)

PROCEDURES AND TECHNIQUES

Diagnosis

This tradition uses all the conventional diagnostic procedures of allopathy in terms of laboratory tests, X rays, and other high-tech procedures. In addition, osteopathic physicians receive training in palpation, the use of touch to assess such factors as tissue texture changes, heat, cold, motion and lack of motion, pain and absence of pain.

A wide range of hands-on methods are used to identify structural problems. According to Holland, "The difference between a real osteopathic physician and an allopathic physician is that we are taught to use our bodies as 'diagnostic instruments' through palpation."

When meeting with a traditional osteopathic physician for the first time, often the patient disrobes to have a full structural exam in addition to the rest of the history. This is a routine part of the physical exam because of the interrelationship between structure and function and is a standard part of osteopathic practice regardless of the specialty of the practitioner. It allows the practitioner to assess the person's posture, motion of limbs, symmetry, and gait while walking. This may entail more time than an allopath ordinarily spends.

Andrew

Andrew, six months old, had a difficult birth, with his head getting stuck. At six weeks he began to arch his back and at three months he was diagnosed with infantile spasms—frequent intractable seizures. He was also diagnosed as cortically blind with a bilateral optic nerve atrophy. His mother was told that he would be in a chronic vegetative state and was advised to institutionalize him.

A friend recommended she bring him to Carlisle Holland, D.O., who found Andrew to have a severely bent cranium. With the help of anticonvulsant medication, Holland was able to work with him weekly for about three months using CranioSacral Therapy™ and other manipulative techniques.

Eventually Holland was able to get the bend out of the back of Andrew's head, at which time his craniosacral mechanism began to pulsate normally and the seizures immediately stopped. Over the next three months he was tapered off the anticonvulsants and has not had a seizure since. He is now four years old.

"We now know that he sees, tracks objects, and looks with both eyes," adds Holland. "He's sitting up and trying to crawl. He is also working with a physical therapist who does Feldenkrais movement integration. If we could not correct the head problem, we would never have gotten him off anticonvulsants."

Treatment

Osteopathic physicians often integrate allopathic drugs with osteopathic manipulation. For example, they may administer antibiotics for pneumonia and, in keeping with the understanding that the rule of the artery is supreme and that the lymphatic system contributes to the healing process, they may accompany this with a manipulative technique called the *lymphatic pump* described below.

According to Yusuf Erskine, D.O., of Sebastopol, California, there are specific techniques for every part of the body, all sharing the purpose of affecting the functioning nervous system, the blood circulation, and the lymphatic circulation. Following are several of the most commonly used approaches.

Lymphatic Pump. Also known as the *thoracic pump* or *rib raising*, this technique manipulates the rib cage and thoracic spine to improve lymph circulation in the chest cavity. The practitioner may place the palms of his or her hands on the patient's chest and rhythmically pump, or may place the hands underneath the patient's back, rhythmically raising them up and down on the treatment table.

By intermittently applying and releasing pressure to the lymphatic system, a vacuumlike pumping action results. The goal is to normalize the structure and increase lymphatic drainage.

Joint Mobilization. This involves the practitioner in gently moving limbs through their range of motion in order to expand the range and to release restrictions.

Muscle Energy Manipulation. In muscle energy techniques the patient pushes or moves a certain way against resistance provided by the physician in order to release a certain holding pattern. The purpose is to extend the range of motion and to correct motion dysfunction. It involves contracting or moving muscles in a precisely controlled direction.

The counterforce applied by the practitioner varies in intensity depending on whether the principle being used is isometric (practitioner equally resisting the patient's force), isotonic (patient overcomes the practitioner's resistance), or isolytic (practitioner overcomes patient's force). The method works to normalize dysfunctional relationships among different muscle

218

groups, often resulting from trauma or injury, that have resulted in structural problems in the body.

Articulatory Techniques (High Velocity-Low Amplitude Thrust Techniques). These methods are similar to those of chiropractic and involve the rapid adjustment of joints throughout the body. Often there is a popping sound caused by vaporization of fluid in the joints as the space within them expands. As Holland explains, "When you ask a joint to expand its volume faster than it can fill with fluid, part of the fluid vaporizes." Stretching the joint capsules suddenly in the spine allows the spinal cord to "reset" its position relative to the spinal joints, thus allowing the nervous system to return to a more normal firing rate and improved biomechanical efficiency of the entire system.

Positioning Techniques. This involves finding a posture or position that allows the patient to gain relief from an injury or trauma by releasing pressure or strain on the injured tissues. It is often used to promote relaxation of muscular spasms.

Myofascial Release. Myofascial techniques are intended to help the body reactivate an area that is restricted. Restrictions in the movement of muscles past each other are caused by loss of lubrication and limitation of gliding motion of the fascia—the flexible envelopelike sheaths that encapsulate muscles and muscle groups. When chronic tension or acute trauma occur, the fascia associated with different muscles or other tissues can become "stuck" or fixed in a position that impedes the smooth, easy movement of the muscles.

Manipulation of the muscles and fascia helps to release these "stuck" places, called "myofascial restrictions." According to Erskine, "If done successfully, the holding pattern dissolves back into the wholeness of the body."

Cranial Manipulation. One of the more dramatic approaches offered by osteopathy involves the subtle manipulation of the bones and tissues of the skull and spine (collectively called the craniosacral system). Work in this field was initiated by William

219

Nicole

Nicole, a six-month-old baby girl, had had colic from birth and had never slept more than an hour and a half. She was the firstborn and had a thirty-six-hour labor. She would draw her legs up and cry like her belly hurt. She was tested for upper GI problems and had X rays of her neck taken, but no cause of her distress was found.

Upon examination Carlisle Holland, D.O., found that her head was pushed down hard on the upper neck on one side and had what is called a condylar compression, where the condyle of the occiput attaches to the neck on the right side. She could only nurse the mother's left breast, could not nurse on the right, and had difficulty suckling well.

Manipulation was used to balance the occiput, take out the compression, and restore the range of motion in her neck so she could rotate her head symmetrically.

Holland reported, "The moment her head became balanced, she gave a huge sigh and went completely relaxed. She then slept fourteen hours. The parents were worried something may be wrong, but when she woke up she was fine. She never went back to the fussing and crying, her sleeping straightened out, and she nursed equally on both breasts. The mother came in the next week and looked ten years younger, and the child was happy."

Treatment was three sessions over a two-week period.

Sutherland, D.O., who developed what he called "osteopathy in the cranial field" or "cranial osteopathy" in the 1930s.

Sutherland observed that the bones of the skull are connected by sutures, much like joints. In fact the head is more a "visco-elastic" or "visco-plastic" structure than a hard bony object. When a child is born the bones are separated, but they later fuse along flexible suture lines. The flexibility of the sutures allows the bones to be manipulated.

Sutherland found that the application of very light finger pressure anywhere in the craniosacral system can influence the pressure and circulation of cerebrospinal fluid throughout. Circulation or drainage of other fluids in the head (including blood, lymph, and sinus fluids) can also be affected by manipulation of the craniosacral system. Finally, he determined that the healthy craniosacral system pulsates at a rate of about six to fifteen times per minute; restoring proper pulsation is often a goal of treatment.

Variations of craniosacral manipulation include sacro-occipital technique (SOT, also called "craniopathy") developed by Major B. DeJarnette, D.C., who studied with Sutherland (see Chapter 8, Chiropractic); and CranioSacral Therapy™ developed by John Upledger, D.O. (not limited to osteopaths and discussed in Chapter 9, Massage Therapy and Bodywork).

Visceral Manipulation. These techniques involve the manual application of subtle pressures to encourage normal mobility and positioning of internal organs and connective tissues. For example, the practitioner can actually touch the gallbladder through the skin and soft tissue. A variation is to use hand pressure to stretch out an area or free up restrictions that are mere inches beyond the practitioner's direct reach.

SCIENTIFIC SUPPORT

The earliest studies in osteopathy focused on establishing the effects of lesions in the spinal column on internal organs and tissues in animals. The noted osteopathic researcher Louisa Burns, D.O., was the first to establish and carry on a long-term research program examining the principles of osteopathic theory. Burns had entered the profession in the late 1800s after recovering from spinal meningitis with the help of osteopathic treatment.

As a result of her two decades of work, in 1927 she wrote:

> Any vertebral lesion causes, in the viscera innervated from the neighboring segments of the spinal cord, certain definite circulatory, nutritional, and functional changes which are invariable and certain in any mammal for the same spinal area, and are invariable for the same animal in different areas of the spinal column. . . . There is a definite and certain pathological picture which is due to a vertebral lesion and to no other condition in its entirety.[6]

The focus of osteopathic research has expanded dramatically over recent decades. In fact, a great deal of the current and recent research deals with the basic biomedical sciences, both with animals and human subjects, and much of it is indistinguishable from that being conducted in allopathic medical schools.

There are, however, also studies on the unique aspects of osteopathic medicine. For example, an interesting study conducted at the Department of Psychiatry, Chicago College of Osteopathic Medicine, with forty-one patients examined whether there were musculoskeletal differences that differentiate psychotic patients from those with affective disorders.

The psychotic patients were found to have significantly more structural dysfunctions in the midcervical region and the lower extremities than those with affective disorders. On the other hand, the latter group had significantly more dysfunction in the thoracic region. The researchers concluded that the structural examination can differentiate between patients with psychotic and affective disorders and that these disorders affect different regions of the spine.[7]

While this tradition has nowhere near the resources of allopathy for research, it is rich with clinical observations and informal studies that obviously confirm osteopathic principles. There have been many studies over the years on the effects of manipulation on neurophysiology, neurochemistry, and the clinical course of many medical conditions, though most have been on a small scale.

As observed by Myron Beal, D.O., a professor at the Michigan State University College of Osteopathic Medicine, "It is important to point out that clinical studies of the effectiveness of manipulation are limited, and most studies are subject to criticism in terms of the research design, controls, use of investigator blinding, types of manipulation, tests of structural diagnosis, skill of the manipulator, and number of treatments given."[8]

Nevertheless, those summarized below give a sampling of findings from the better clinical studies of manipulation.

Musculoskeletal Problems

Low Back Pain. A 1992 study examined the effects of osteopathic manipulation on the lumbar vertebra in twenty-six people. The technique used was high velocity–low amplitude manipulation, which was found to decrease EMG activity (a measure of muscular tension) during movement and also to relieve low back pain and muscle spasm.[9]

A 1971 study examined the effects of manipulation on forty-seven patients with symptoms of lumbar nerve root compression. Seven patients had conservative care without manipulation, nineteen had surgery, and twenty-one had manipulation while under anesthesia. The researchers concluded that manipulation under anesthesia produced lasting improvement in those patients whose condition was not severe enough to show visible evidence of nerve root compression by electromyography (EMG). Those with more severe symptoms, however, had only temporary improvement.[10]

Headache. A study of patients with muscle contraction headaches in 1979 divided patients into four groups: palpatory examination with manipulation, palpatory examination alone, manipulation alone, or rest in a supine position. The group receiving the combination of palpation and manipulation had significantly less pain than the other three groups.[11]

Myofibrositis and Herniated Disc. A 1963 study of the effects of manipulation conducted under anesthesia found a favorable response to the therapy in 96.3 percent of patients with myofibrositis and in 70.7 percent of patients with herniated disc. However, since 51 percent of those with herniated disc required surgery, the study concluded the benefits were transient for that group.[12]

Peripheral Nerve Problems. A double-blind clinical trial was conducted on the effects of manipulative treatment for 197 patients with peripheral nerve complaints. In 167 patients, treatment of a specific area of the spine produced a therapeutic response associated with improvement in skin temperature of the affected limb.[13,14]

Shoulder Function in the Elderly. A study examined the effects of osteopathic manipulation on the shoulder joints in twenty-nine elderly patients (over sixty-two years old) with chronic shoulder pain, decreased range of motion, or decreased functional abilities in one shoulder. Significant improvement in range of motion was found.[15]

Fibromyalgia. One study measured the effects of manipulation on tender points in eighteen patients with fibromyalgia syndrome. Six treatments were provided, one to three weeks apart. Results included reduction in tender point pain and improved daily functioning.[16]

Another study compared the pain levels in patients receiving manipulation, manipulation accompanied by self-help training, and moist heat only. Both groups receiving the manipulation had significantly less pain and those with the self-help training improved further.[17]

In another study, nineteen patients were treated with manipulation for generalized muscle pain, fatigue, nonrestorative sleep, and multiple tender points. Sixteen reported improved sleep and eighteen reported subjective pain relief. Most had significant reductions of tender points after weekly manipulation for four weeks. Four patients had less than eleven tender points after the study and thus no longer fulfilled the diagnostic criteria for fibromyalgia. The effects of the treatment lasted an average of 3.7 weeks.[18]

Lung Problems

Pneumonia in the Elderly. A study of the use of manipulative therapy in hospitalized elderly patients undergoing antibiotic therapy for pneumonia found that those receiving manipulation required significantly less antibiotic treatment and had significantly shorter hospital stays.[19]

Asthmatic Bronchitis. In 1925 a study was conducted on the effects of manipulative treatment for twenty patients with asthmatic bronchitis. Results included a 50 percent decrease in asthma attacks for half the patients.[20] A 1957 study of twenty patients also found decreased need for medication after manipulative treatment.[21]

Chronic Obstructive Lung Disease. A 1975 study of the effects of manipulation in seventeen patients with chronic obstructive lung disease found significant improvement in pulmonary CO^2 levels, oxygen saturation, total lung capacity, and residual volume.[22] A 1982 study of a hundred patients with upper, middle, or pararespiratory illness concluded that manipulation limited the duration of illness, relieved symptoms, and prevented complications and recurrences.[23]

Childhood Infections

Measles. A 1962 study tracked 204 children with measles who were given manipulative therapy. Only thirty-one had complications and of these only seven were considered of a serious nature.[24] A 1966 study reviewed 4600 cases in which manipulative therapy was used for upper respiratory infections. The complication rate found was 16.9 percent, far below the 33- to 50-percent complication rate associated with the standard allopathic treatment of the time.[25]

Respiratory Infections. The effectiveness of manipulative therapy and antibiotics in respiratory infections were compared in a 1965 study of 252 infants and children. Those who received the combination of treatments recovered faster then those receiving either therapy alone.[26]

Hypertension

A 1961 study of the effects of manipulation on hypertension in a hundred patients found an average drop in blood pressure of 33/9 (i.e., average reduction from 199/123 to 166/114).[27]

STRENGTHS AND LIMITATIONS

The greatest strength of osteopathic medicine is its versatility. Practitioners are able to use all the methods of allopathy including pharmaceutical drugs, surgery, emergency medicine, acute care, and hospitalization while also being able to offer osteopathic manipulation. In addition, many use other alternative practices.

Although formal research is not as plentiful as it could be, clinical experience has found this tradition particularly effective with musculoskeletal problems including fibromyalgia syndrome, arthritis, rheumatism, spinal and joint disorders, chronic pain, stress or trauma, pregnancy discomfort, and injuries from work, sports, and motor vehicle accidents. Essentially any condition that involves muscular or skeletal features can benefit from such manipulation. Manipulation offers some real advantages over drugs in that it is able to achieve many of the same outcomes with no side effects or concerns about drug interaction.

The fact that manipulation involves a great deal of hands-on contact by the physician is of great importance to many people. The contact helps patients feel a caring personal connection with the physician.

One unique strength is that osteopathic surgeons encourage the use of manipulation postoperatively. They were among the first to advocate early ambulation because they recognized that the body is more likely to deteriorate rapidly if it is immobile, as is often the case with extended periods of recovery from surgery.

Historically, patients receiving major surgery have been confined to bed for weeks. In the osteopathic perspective, such an approach works against the body's abilities to heal itself. Hence early ambulation is advocated to enhance healing. Osteopathic surgeons may use rib raising or even passive motion of body parts to stimulate the nervous system, lymphatic flow, and blood circulation.

Carlisle Holland, D.O., offers the following perspective:

We have the advantage of knowing medicine, so we can be critical while looking at situations clinically and looking at alternatives. We know ways to get around medication or avoid surgery and do it in a way that is responsible. We know the consequences, and we know medicines and their power.

If we choose to avoid prescribing medicine or to do homeopathy, we do it from a solid grounding in medicine and in understanding the musculoskeletal system. We have the best of all worlds.

227

This tradition has many of the same limitations as allopathy in that the more advanced a chronic or degenerative illness is, particularly cancer, the less effective it is in reversing a disease process.

THE PRACTITIONER-PATIENT RELATIONSHIP

Osteopathic theory holds that the therapeutic potency of the physician-patient relationship plays a key role in healing. The physician has a role as a healer and is thought of as a facilitator of healing. Medicine cannot be practiced in a void but in the context of this therapeutic interpersonal relationship.

The fact that all the manipulative modalities are hands-on approaches enhances the rapport between the physician and patient. As mentioned earlier, the initial exam may take longer than that of an allopathic practitioner because of the structural exam. Subsequent office visits tend also to take longer because of the emphasis on structural exam and hands-on treatment.

It should be remembered that osteopathic physicians vary in the degree to which they align themselves with the traditional osteopathic perspective versus that of allopathy. The patient can determine the approach used by a particular practitioner by asking whether manipulation is used and how much time is scheduled for office visits.

EVALUATING PERSONAL RESULTS

Outcomes of treatment can be measured by conventional laboratory tests, palpation of the spine or other parts of the body by the physician (using his or her hands to feel changes in the body), and manipulation to determine changes in the range of motion of joints.

Those practicing craniosacral manipulation can also detect changes in the craniosacral motion and craniosacral pulse as indications of changes in structure and function.

As with any other tradition, ultimately the subjective response of the patient is the most important criterion.

RELATIONSHIP TO OTHER FORMS OF MEDICINE

Osteopathic medicine is among the most versatile of all traditions. It contains a wide diversity of practitioners who integrate the full range of other traditions in their practice as well as those who are more narrowly specialized along the lines of allopathy.

Practitioners who follow the allopathic model of office practice, with the average consultation time of twelve to fifteen minutes per office visit, are less likely to provide the more vitalistically oriented forms of health care. If you are seeking a vitalistic orientation, it may make more sense to accompany treatment by this tradition with that of another.

The practices of the majority of osteopathic physicians can be supported in a complementary way by most other traditions. Obviously, the only potential areas of duplication would be with allopathy, chiropractic, and certain forms of bodywork, so concurrent treatment by those may not be appropriate.

COSTS

The costs of office visits with an osteopathic physician are generally the same as those of allopathy and insurance coverage is also the same. There may be slightly lower fees in rural areas.

Overall treatment costs may be lower if the practitioner relies more on manipulation than pharmaceuticals or technological treatments. Many practitioners choose this tradition because of its orientation toward prevention and less invasive treatments, which are usually lower in cost.

CHOOSING A PRACTITIONER

Since all osteopathic physicians are fully licensed, the main considerations in choosing one are whether you are seeking a specialist or a general practitioner and whether you are interested in manipulative treatment.

Specialties will be named with any physician's literature about his or her practice. As for the use of manipulation, you can simply ask when calling the office whether that practitioner uses it. Another way to assess expertise in manipulation is membership in the American Academy of Osteopathy (see below).

Organizations

American Osteopathic Association (AOA) is the primary professional association for this tradition. It has several departments and bureaus to coordinate medical education, research, legislative advocacy, public education, and the advancement of the profession. Address: 142 East Ontario St., Chicago, IL 60611, phone (312) 280–5800.

The American Academy of Osteopathy (AAO) is a subgroup of physicians within the AOA who are actively using manipulative medicine in their practice. They offer board certification in osteopathic manipulative medicine. The academy has two thousand members who elect to use manipulation as a primary modality of treatment. Address: 3500 DePauw Blvd., Suite 1080, Indianapolis, IN 46268–1136, phone (317) 879–1881.

The Cranial Academy teaches cranial manipulation in the

tradition developed by William Sutherland, D.O. The academy has over eight hundred members and provides local referrals to trained practitioners. Address: 3500 DePauw Blvd., Indianapolis, IN 46268, phone (317) 879–0713.

CHAPTER 8

CHIROPRACTIC: OPENING THE GATES

"A patient finally went to a chiropractor for her back pain after finding no relief with the orthopedist. After three adjustments and a week of no symptoms, she had a follow-up visit with her M.D. Upon learning about the success of the D.C., the orthopedist stated, 'That was just the placebo effect.' The patient responded, 'If it works so well, why didn't you use it?' "
—ROBERT MOOTZ, D.C.[1]

Chiropractors represent the second largest group of primary care providers in the United States after physicians, with 45,000 practitioners, and they receive two-thirds of all health care visits for back pain.[2] The growing demand for this tradition is revealed by three observations reported in the Eisenberg study that was published in *The New England Journal of Medicine* in January 1993.

First, back problems are the most frequently reported ailment for which alternative therapies are sought. Second, of all the unconventional therapies examined for all health concerns, chiropractic was second only to mind/body medicine in frequency of use. Third, the total number of people using chiropractic is now estimated at 10 percent of the population[3]—double that reported in 1980.[4]

Origins

In the fall of 1895, a janitor named Harvey Lillard entered the office of a popular, eccentric healer named D. D. Palmer in Davenport, Iowa. Palmer was practicing at a time prior to the advent of licensing laws for physicians in that state and when many doctors, particularly in the Midwest, had no formal medical education. A self-taught student of anatomy and physiology, he was known as a successful faith healer and practitioner of magnetic healing and the laying on of hands.

Lillard, the maintenance man for Palmer's office building, had been deaf since straining himself seventeen years earlier while working in a cramped position. Upon examining the man, Palmer discovered a painful prominent vertebra in the upper spine, which Lillard confirmed had been the source of the original injury that had led to his deafness. As the story goes, Palmer applied a sharp thrust, repositioning the bone, and Lillard's hearing returned better than ever. Thus chiropractic was born.

Manipulation of the spine had been a part of the healing repertoires of virtually all traditional cultures, from the ancient Greeks to the Pacific islanders to the Native Americans. However, Palmer pioneered a modern theory of joint-oriented nerve interference that quickly brought adherents at a time when interest in natural medicine was booming (naturopathy and osteopathy were also developing about this time).

He named this approach chiropractic, combining the Greek *cheir* (hand) and *praxis* (practice). The first chiropractic college was formed by Palmer in 1897. The first state licensing law for chiropractic was passed in 1913.

In his early writings, Palmer's original philosophy described this approach as a means of connecting "man the spiritual" to "man the physical" by eliminating interference to the flow of "Innate Intelligence" through each individual. This Innate Intelligence, a somewhat elusive, almost metaphysical phenomenon, flows through the nervous system. The clearer the nervous sys-

233

tem is, the more the Innate Intelligence can express itself and fully enliven the person's body and organs.

Palmer's fascination with Innate Intelligence and its relationship to the nervous system formed the basis of his theory. Chiropractic's origins really had little to do with backaches, headaches, or neck aches. The theory held that any disease process anywhere in the body is affected at least in part by the ability of the nervous system to enervate and enliven that area. Hence, any disease process can potentially benefit from chiropractic.

Turf Wars

This tradition had a rocky relationship with conventional medicine until only recently. Palmer's son B. J., who took the role of being the tradition's most vocal salesman, did not exactly foster an amicable relationship with his public declaration that "D.C. equals disease conquered; M.D. equals more dope—more death."

Antipathy grew until the 1960s when the American Medical Association officially declared to its own membership that it was unethical for any of them to associate with any member of "the cult of chiropractic." The AMA's Committee on Quackery, formed in 1963, was charged with the purpose of debunking the chiropractic tradition.

In 1976, Chester Wilk and four fellow chiropractors filed a federal suit against the AMA, the American Hospital Association, and six other medical associations, charging them with antitrust violations by conspiring to eliminate chiropractic and by refusal to associate professionally with chiropractors. Their victory in this suit in 1987 was a milestone in the acceptance and legitimization of this tradition.

Walter

Walter was a forty-two-year-old engineer experiencing insomnia, anxiety attacks, night sweats, numbing and tingling in his hands and feet, marginal hypertension, and chronic fatigue. He had been given numerous diagnoses and was taking a heavy tranquilizer. He sought chiropractic for low pack pain and headache.

He was found to have a very high respiration rate (twenty-two breaths per minute, normal is twelve to fourteen), indicating chronic hyperventilation.

After five spinal adjustments over a ten-day period he reported sleeping normally for the first time in ten years. The outcomes included normalization of respiration rate and blood pressure and cessation of anxiety attacks, insomnia, fatigue, back pain, and headaches. According to his practitioner, James Adams, D.C., of Sonoma, California, "The release of subluxations caused all these beneficial changes. He has some patterns that will recur and will require periodic attention, but essentially it has dramatically changed his quality of life."

Chiropractic Education

The profession has experienced rather phenomenal growth in the number of practitioners since the 1980s and most chiropractic colleges operate at maximum enrollment. There are fourteen colleges in the United States accredited by the Council on Chiropractic Education (CCE), one each in Canada and England, and two in Australia. The CCE is the sole accrediting organization recognized by the U.S. Department of Education.

Admission to a chiropractic college requires at least two years of undergraduate study with course work in biology and chemistry but does not require a bachelor's degree (between a third and half have undergraduate degrees or higher prior to chiropractic training[5]). The chiropractic curriculum requires four years full-time study with a minimum of 4200 hours of course work.

Many of the textbooks are the same as those used in allopathic medical schools. The curriculum includes anatomy; biochemistry; physiology; microbiology; pathology; public health; physical, clinical, and laboratory diagnosis; gynecology; obstetrics; pediatrics; geriatrics; dermatology; otolaryngology; roentgenology (X ray); psychology; dietetics; orthopedics; physical therapy; first aid and emergency medicine; spinal analysis; principles and practice of chiropractic; adjustive technique; and research methods and procedure.

KEY PRINCIPLES

The Vitalistic Principle

An important philosophical underpinning of chiropractic is the vitalistic principle, which holds that the human organism can keep itself healthy if there are no barriers to full expression of all its vital functions. The body has the ability to heal itself from within.

Furthermore, the life force (or Innate Intelligence, as Palmer referred to it) emanates throughout the body through the nervous system. In a sense, the nervous system is thought of as the conduit of the life force. By manipulating the spine and other joints through which the nervous system passes (the spine itself is a series of joints), chiropractors see themselves as removing barriers or obstacles to the full expression of this life force, thereby allowing the functioning necessary for health.

The vitalistic model distinguishes chiropractic from the conventional medical model in that chiropractors do not directly treat disease but rather facilitate the body's own restorative

236

powers. The concept of vital force has of course eluded scientific measurement. Like *chi* in Chinese medicine, *prana* in Ayurveda, and the vital force in homeopathy, it is a major premise of chiropractic whose truth is self-evident to the practitioner.

Holism

Another important principle is the notion of holism, the recognition that the body is a network of systems all interpenetrating and influencing one another. Within this context, the nervous system is the master system in the sense that it mediates the functioning of all other systems to at least some degree. Hence any obstacle to perfect function of the nervous system has potentially far-reaching effects and chiropractic's focal point of concern is the integrity of the nervous system.[6]

The Focus of Treatment: Subluxation

The term "subluxation" actually means "less than full dislocation" in a joint comprised of two vertebra. In other words, there is a malalignment or dislocation of the vertebra in the joint, but not so severe as to be a complete dislocation. Such subluxations occur normally in the minor bumps and accidents of everyday life.

The basis of chiropractic theory is that subluxations alter the normal neurophysiologic functioning in the person. D. D. Palmer coined the term to describe a misalignment of vertebra that results in undue pressure on the spinal cord or nerves. Another term sometimes used to describe this condition is "segmental dysfunction," referring to a segment of the spine.

To Palmer a subluxation was a joint problem in the spine in which the flow of Innate Intelligence is disturbed or impeded.

Norma

Norma is sixty-nine. She came after having surgery on her low back for the relief of tingling. She had extensive osteoarthritis (degenerative changes in the spine). After the surgery the symptoms did not abate and seemed to be worsening.

She was also being treated for congestive heart failure and hypertension, experienced dizziness, and had edema. Her hands and feet were cold. She used to crochet, but all her control movements were being affected.

She was seen three times per week for four weeks, then twice per week for four weeks. After that the frequency of visits continued to reduce over several months, to where she is now seen about once a month. In the first four weeks she lost fourteen pounds of fluid from her entire body, a great deal of which was in her legs.

As James Adams, D.C., explains, "We increased the efficiency of the exchange level at the lungs and we changed the pH factor that influences the ability of the body to process fluids. This loss of fluid from the system remarkably improved the heart." Her blood pressure was reduced by twenty-five points on the systolic and ten points on the diastolic and her requirements for medication dropped significantly.

The inappropriate pressure on nerves (nerve "reflex") caused by subluxation is what causes disturbance in the bodily functions supplied by those nerves and can make the person more vulnerable to disease processes.

According to Larry Oberstein, D.C., of Santa Rosa, California, "What we do as chiropractors is look for interferences in the nervous system in the form of subluxations and remove those interferences to allow the nervous system to function at a higher level. And in the process of functioning at a higher level, the body will begin to heal itself."[7]

The Role of the Musculoskeletal System

The musculoskeletal system and the viscera or internal organs can in a sense be thought of as two sides of the same coin. Of course they are interdependent, but there can be different points of view about the nature of their relationship.

The traditional chiropractic view expressed by the "straights" ("straight chiropractic" will be discussed later) is that biological function is a manifestation of living structure. Any disturbance in structure causes a corresponding disturbance in function. Vertebral subluxation is a disturbance in the structural relationship of the vertebra and the nerves they protect, which reduces the body's ability to maintain its own health.[8]

William Meeker, D.C., dean of research at Palmer College of Chiropractic-West in San Jose, California, and president of the Consortium of Chiropractic Research, offers an interesting insight to the chiropractic perspective:

> Some people think the bones and muscles are there to carry the heart and lungs, but we see it the other way around. We like to say that the viscera is there to support the musculoskeletal system, to make sure it works right and allows us to be mobile on the earth. Most of the body is really taken up by the bones, joints, and muscles, not by the heart, lungs, and gut.[9]

And in the words of John Pammer, D.C., president of the American Chiropractic Association, "We categorize ourselves as mechanical engineers, while medical doctors are chemical engineers."[10]

The Causes of Illness

This tradition holds that much of illness occurs as a result of disturbances in the nervous system. Such disturbances are caused by derangements of the musculoskeletal structure and they may cause or aggravate disease in various parts or functions of the body.

Subluxations occur as a normal part of living in any culture. However, from an anthropological perspective our bodies were not designed to sit for long periods of time. The modern sedentary lifestyle consisting of little exercise and long periods of sitting, either at desks, in cars, or at home, puts an unnatural strain on the spine and contributes to subluxations. The spine does not receive the degree of daily movement with which it evolved. Modern lifestyles often impede a normal, healthful degree of flexibility.

Many chiropractors also hold that health is further compromised by other aspects of lifestyle, such as inadequate nutrition as a result of the processing and denaturing of foods and pollution and chronic stress, which add further to the burden on the body. All these factors together create a situation in which the flow of vital force through the nervous system is impaired at a time when it is needed to be at its optimum; hence the plethora of chronic and degenerative illnesses we face today.

VARIATIONS WITHIN THE TRADITION

The vast majority of chiropractors are generalists who do not have specialized certification. However there are a variety of specializations available through extensive postgraduate training programs, some of which require up to three years of study.

Board certifications are offered by the ACA in radiology, orthopedics, sports injuries, nutrition, internal medicine, and neurology. (Their designations are described later in the section on Choosing a Practitioner.)

"Straights" and "Mixers"

There is no universal agreement about what categories might be meaningful in describing varieties of chiropractic. One approach that has been used in the past, though it vastly oversimplifies matters, is the dichotomy of "straight" and "mixer." These terms have been used to describe the degree to which a practitioner limits practice to what is historically unique about chiropractic as opposed to including modalities and concepts used by other medical traditions.

A minority of practitioners, about 15 percent, call themselves "straight" chiropractors. They define straight chiropractic as "a limited, primary health care profession" with "responsibility and authority . . . limited to the anatomy of the spine and immediate articulations, the condition of vertebral subluxation, and a scope of practice which encompasses addressing vertebral subluxations as well as educating patients and advising them about subluxations."[11]

This group holds that in communication with patients, practitioners should not use terms used by other health traditions. For example, they prefer "analysis" to "diagnosis" and "adjustment" to "manipulation." They also oppose use of the terms "treatment," "chiropractic medicine," and "chiropractic physician."

The term "mixer" was coined by advocates of straight chiropractic to describe those whose practice extends beyond the narrow focus on vertebral subluxation. They use a wider range of modalities as well as concepts from diverse health care traditions in their practice.

This is actually the majority of practitioners. Many integrate methods from other traditions, the most common adjunct being nutritional supplementation. For some, however, their entire practice has evolved away from the use of traditionally chiropractic modalities and toward a greater focus on another tradition. Their licensure as a primary care provider gives them the freedom to employ these other modalities at their discretion.

There are D.C.s who integrate Chinese medicine, Ayurveda, naturopathy, homeopathy, massage or bodywork, mind/body approaches, or other healing methods. Individuals often develop their own unique reputation and synthesis of different traditions.

"Subluxation-Based" and "Medically Oriented"

Another point of view on the varieties of practice is offered by Terry Rondberg, D.C., president of the World Chiropractic Alliance. He sees a distinction emerging between those who are "subluxation-based" and those who are "medically oriented."

In his view, subluxation-based chiropractors are those who use spinal adjustment as the heart of their practice, whether or not they use other modalities from other medical traditions. They maintain allegiance to the original principle of Innate Intelligence as being the key factor in healing.

Medically oriented chiropractors, which Rondberg estimates at 20 percent of the profession, constitute a growing number of practitioners whose thinking takes a more allopathic perspective in terms of the diagnosis and treatment of disease. They are also more liberal in terms of using allopathic-type procedures in their practice.

Rondberg notes that in some states chiropractors are allowed to perform minor surgery and deliver babies. He cites the variety of board certifications now offered by the ACA as evidence of a movement toward a "medicalization" of chiropractic or a greater alignment of it with allopathic thinking.

According to Meeker, the real issues in the dialogue over

Ronnie

Ronnie, a seven-year-old boy, had developed eczema as an infant in the creases of the arms and elbows and occasionally in the armpits. At age five he began to develop some allergies and bronchial asthma. In acute periods his areas of eczema would be weeping, crusty, and cracked. He was taking bronchial dilators and during severe episodes he would take steroids.

He would miss long periods of school and at one time had missed four and a half months with recurring problems of both the asthma and eczema.

Under chiropractic care he was seen three times a week for four weeks, then twice a week for six weeks, followed by longer intervals between adjustments. Now at age nine he is seen once a month. Only 2 to 3 percent of the eczema remains, he has no more of the wheezing asthmatic episodes, and he uses no medication.

James Adams, D.C., explains, "Ronnie had problems in the lower cervical and lower thoracic regions. These affected the dilatory capability and sensitivity in the bronchial areas and the regulatory centers in the brain stem. The eczema and the asthma are both coming from the same problem—an overactive immune response. He remains a little sensitive to certain environmental agents and his skin is still a little on the dry side."

the varieties within the tradition are the scope of practice and responsibility. "The truth is that most chiropractors are willing to take responsibility for the diagnosis (they are trained to do so in all accredited chiropractic colleges) and the triage of patients to appropriate care. Most will admit—and this is borne out by actual survey data—that chiropractic therapeutic expertise is best suited for neuromusculoskeletal complaints in which joint subluxation plays a role."[12]

Network Chiropractic

This is an approach that has been developing since 1979 by Donald Epstein, D.C. It draws upon chiropractic's traditional adjustment techniques and works with the body's Innate Intelligence. Its uniqueness lies in its use of a unified system of twelve techniques with special attention to their timing and sequencing.

PROCEDURES AND TECHNIQUES

Chiropractic is a drugless and nonsurgical approach. Hands-on physical manipulation of the musculoskeletal system is the primary means of treatment. This can include all muscles and joints, but the greatest emphasis is on those of the back.

Before Treatment

Before the initial consultation some practitioners send out medical history questionnaires in advance and even audiotapes for orientation purposes.

Following the history, a physical examination may be given, the extent of which will depend on the presenting problem. Chiropractors are trained to conduct a standard physical exam the same as a conventional physician. State laws vary as to whether standard physical exams by a chiropractor are considered acceptable for legal purposes.

The exam allows an assessment of the appropriateness of the case and then a treatment plan is devised. Further assessment can include measuring leg length, muscle tone, heel tension, adduction stress, microwave radiation on the body, palpation (how the body and the vertebra feel), and instrumentation.

Therapies

Physiotherapy. Physiotherapy includes electrical stimulation, ice, heat, ultrasound, and traction. Electrical stimulation involves placing a pad on an area of the body in order to introduce an electrical current. It may be used for a form of deep tissue massage or to help pump exidates (body fluid) from the tissue around a sprain to relieve the edema (swelling or fluid) that has built up around it.

Ice may be used for pain control and heat for sedation. Ultrasound is a form of micromassage that directs sound vibrations into the tissue to stimulate circulation or remove toxins, edema, and electrolytes that have built up around an injury. This is especially useful in frozen shoulder, bursitis, and tendinitis.

Traction is conducted in a variety of ways to stretch or lengthen the spine and relieve pressure on subluxations.

Most chiropractors will also use various forms of soft tissue manipulation, trigger point manipulation, or direct deep tissue massage.

Adjustments. The adjustment has been traditionally defined as a high velocity—low amplitude thrust that lasts about a tenth of a second. This means the practitioner quickly applies a small, highly controlled force to the body in an effort to remove subluxations. The purpose of all adjustments is to restore normal joint function, which should be immediately evident by improved mobility.

Done properly, the procedures are painless. There is usually an audible snapping or popping sound, which signifies that tiny gas bubbles that have built up within the fluid-filled space in the joint as a result of its immobility have been released.

There are two general kinds of spinal adjustment. "Nonspecific long-lever manipulations" involve placing the femur (thighbone), shoulder, head, or pelvis in various positions to manipulate the entire spine as a whole unit. "Short-lever spinal adjustments" use hands-on pressure on or near a specific vertebra to move a particular vertebral joint.

There are a variety of special tables that can be used to help the practitioner position the patient in such a way as to more easily access certain joints and move them within a certain plane.

Other Manipulations. Beyond the adjustments described above, a variety of other manipulations may be used to help restore full freedom of motion in joints and to loosen fixations or adhesions that may have occurred in the surrounding tissues as a result of immobility. This includes stretching, traction, and slow manipulations that may be applied after a condition has been treated with physiotherapy and has healed.

Many chiropractors also use cranial manipulation, which has been a part of the tradition's repertoire for many years. One of this century's earlier chiropractors, Dr. Major B. DeJarnette of Omaha, Nebraska, studied with the osteopath William Sutherland, D.O., who developed cranial osteopathy in the 1930s. DeJarnette coined the terms "craniopathy" and "sacro-occipital technique (SOT)" for his variety of manipulation.

According to Robert Dubin, D.C., chiropractic involves manipulation of all of the joints and articulations of the skeleton, so that every joint in the body is an appropriate venue for the chiropractor to address—including those of the skull.

Network chiropractic uses lighter, more subtle touch than people commonly associate with chiropractic. The practitioner may tap lightly on points where the vertebra attach to the meningeal sheath that covers the spinal cord. According to Epstein,

"Most chiropractors go for bone crunching. We only do those type of adjustments after we've released all the tension from the spine and there is still a lack of recovery from a structural or physical trauma."[13]

Follow-Up Care

Increasingly, postural guidelines and lifestyle counseling are part of chiropractic consultation. Patients with serious back problems are also referred to educational programs where they are taught therapeutic exercises. Psychotherapy is sometimes appropriate to aid in coping with necessary behavioral or lifestyle changes to promote recovery.

SCIENTIFIC SUPPORT

Like some other healing traditions, chiropractic has not historically emphasized academic or scientific research. It has been outside the loop of government or private sector funding since it does not use drugs or surgery and is not aligned with major academic institutions.

This is another tradition whose evolution has been based more on art than science, more on the subjective experience of the patient than on objective criteria. Indeed, many of its key concepts are highly theoretical, though their proponents believe in them passionately.

The research climate has changed in recent years with the increasing emphasis on measurable outcomes, cost-effectiveness, and health care reform. The tradition has undertaken to meet the challenge of more rigorous scientific scrutiny by launching several research efforts.

One result is the creation of the Consortium for Chiropractic

OAM-Funded Study

The Office of Alternative Medicine, National Institutes of Health, funded one study related to chiropractic in its initial set of research grants.

Martin Krag of the University of Vermont, Burlington, is developing the technology to measure the severity of restrictions in vertebral motion in lateral bending, axial rotation, and extension and the biomechanical response of the lumbar spine to chiropractic manipulation. His work aims to help measure the amount of force needed to move the vertebra and a five-point scale of the severity of restriction will be developed.

Research, which was established in 1985. This is a nonprofit organization consisting of twenty-six chiropractic colleges, state chiropractic associations, professional societies, and insurance companies. The consortium and the ACA's Foundation for Chiropractic Education and Research have provided increasing leadership in developing the scientific basis of the profession.

Studies currently under way at various colleges include documenting the effects of chiropractic care on head, neck, and shoulder pain; migraine headaches; carpal tunnel syndrome; dysmenorrhea; infant colic; and backache associated with pregnancy.

Immune-Related Conditions

One interesting area of research is in treatment of otitis media (middle ear infection) in children. A study is being conducted that compares the outcomes of medical treatment and chiropractic treatment. While it is not complete, preliminary findings suggest that the chiropractic adjustment seems to have a significant beneficial effect.

The possible mechanisms of action are thought to be either enhanced nerve supply to the inner ear or enhanced immune functioning as a result of the adjustment, but these remain to be further studied. These findings are consistent, however, with many anecdotal reports over the years of enhanced recoveries for otitis media, colds, and other immune-related conditions.

A controlled study that may begin to address such effects was conducted by a team of researchers at the National College of Chiropractic in Lombard, Illinois, and published in the *Journal of Manipulative and Physiological Therapeutics.*[14] Ninety-nine chiropractic students were randomly assigned to one of three groups: sham spinal manipulation (fake adjustment), thoracic spinal manipulation, and soft tissue manipulation.

The researchers measured blood levels of substance P, an important chemical that stimulates immune functioning, and monocyte (an immune cell) responsiveness before and after the procedures. Results indicated significant increases in substance P and monocyte responsiveness for those who received the adjustment. While the findings do not address the question of whether the effects could be clinically significant in the case of a disease process, they do indicate that pathways of influence exist between spinal manipulation and immune functioning.

Another possible mechanism of such effects is that spinal maladjustment may cause the stress response on a chronic basis in the body, thereby indirectly resulting in suppressed immunity. If this is the case and if adjustment relieves that state of chronic stress, then this could help explain positive effects of manipulation on immune-related conditions. A third scenario could be that the adjustment somehow induces the relaxation response, which is also known to enhance immune function.

Obviously research on many aspects of chiropractic is in its early stages. Currently the strongest areas of research are in treatment of low back pain, studies of patient satisfaction with chiropractic care, and cost-effectiveness. The best evidence in these areas is summarized below.

Treatment of Low Back Pain

While low back pain is one of the most common ailments brought to all primary care health providers, it is a condition for which allopathy does not have readily effective conservative treatments. Fortunately, the consensus is that in 90 percent of cases involving uncomplicated back pain symptoms subside within two to twelve weeks whether or not any treatment is used.

The issue for most people of course is whether recovery can be speeded in any way. Today spinal manipulation is one of the few conservative treatments for low back pain that have been found effective, albeit to a modest degree, in randomized trials.

In 1983 a review of literature on conservative treatments was published in the *Journal of the American Medical Association*. It concluded that there is stronger evidence for the short-term efficacy of spinal manipulation than for most other commonly used conservative treatments.[15]

Ironically, the demonstrated *in*effectiveness of some widely used allopathic treatments, such as corticosteroid injections[16] and transcutaneous electrical nerve stimulation,[17] lends indirect support to chiropractic by virtue of the need to examine other options.

Further support is offered by a study published in the *British Medical Journal*. It compared chiropractic and conventional treatment in the British health care system, including traction and various kinds of physical therapy. It found that chiropractic patients demonstrated a greater reduction in pain and disability than those receiving conventional care and the results were maintained beyond two years.[18]

In 1992 a review of research on spinal manipulation for the treatment of low back pain was published in the *Annals of Internal Medicine*. A team of researchers from The Rand Corporation, the UCLA schools of medicine and public health, the Department of Veterans' Affairs Medical Center in West Los Angeles, the Consortium for Chiropractic Research, and Value Health Sciences, Los Angeles, conducted the review.[19]

Ellen

Ellen is eighty-one. She sought chiropractic as a result of headache, neck pain, low back sciatic pain, and vertigo. She also had bladder leakage and had been wearing diapers for five years.

Her diagnosis was cervical spondylosis arthrosis (a degenerative condition in the cervical vertebra). She was treated three times a week for four weeks, then twice a week for four weeks, and is now seen once or twice a month.

Her symptoms have diminished as a result of treatment. She has regained bowel and bladder control and no longer needs diapers.

As James Adams, D.C., explains such degenerative conditions are largely due to inactivity, all too common as we age. "If a joint is fixed in one position any longer than twelve hours," he states, "degenerative forces come into play. That's why at least every twelve hours one must move. When you splint people and put them in casts to fix a fracture, the biggest rehabilitation is not to do with the fracture, it is the joint fixation.

"In my opinion, the pathways that lead to the bowel and bladder control are affected by degenerative changes that take place in the cervical spine. If people were more aware of this they would be far more conscientious about exercise routines and earlier intervention that would prevent the degenerative process."

Twenty-five controlled clinical trials of lumbar spinal manipulation were evaluated in this study. The project took the form of a metanalysis, which is a scientific way of interpreting the collective findings of multiple research studies.

After evaluating the outcomes of all twenty-five studies, the reviewers concluded that patients with uncomplicated, acute low back pain have a 17-percent greater likelihood of recovery within three weeks with spinal manipulation than without it. Since recovery without treatment is estimated at about 50 percent, this means that such manipulation increases the probability of recovery at three weeks by about a third.

Patients with low pain and sciatic nerve irritation were found to be 10 percent more likely to recover at four weeks with such manipulation than without it.

The researchers concluded that spinal manipulation is of short-term benefit for some patients, particularly those with uncomplicated, acute low back pain. They also concluded that there is not sufficient data to determine its effectiveness for chronic low back pain.

In the same article, the authors reported that the risk of serious complication following lumbar manipulation could be estimated at less than one case per 100 million manipulations.

Surgery and Low Back Pain

A 1984 study of a normal healthy sample of people found that 40 percent of those over forty years of age had disk herniations, *but with no pain or other symptoms.*[20] This research found support in a 1994 study published in the prestigious *New England Journal of Medicine*, in which magnetic resonance imaging (MRI) was used to examine the spines of ninety-eight men and women with no back pain. Nearly two thirds were found to have spinal abnormalities including bulging or protruding disks, herniated disks, and degenerated disks.

The researchers concluded, "Given the high prevalence of these findings and of back pain, the discovery by MRI of bulges or protrusions in people with low back pain may frequently be coincidental."[21]

These findings reinforce the fact that we really do not know the exact cause of low back pain, and that many—perhaps most—surgeries for disk abnormalities may be unnecessary. At the heart of this issue is whether the back pain is caused by a problem in the *structure* of the spine, or in the *functioning* of the spine. As the above-mentioned studies suggest, structural abnormalities are not necessarily tied to problems in functioning. The chiropractic perspective is that most problems are *functional*, and conservative responses such as manipulation, exercise, and even watchful waiting are followed by relief because they allow restoration of proper functioning.

According to Dr. John Froymeyer, director of the McClure Musculoskeletal Research Center at the University of Vermont, Americans have ten times more back surgery than people in other Western nations.[22] Furthermore, the Agency for Health Care Policy and Research recently concluded, after a review of four thousand studies, that the expensive tests and therapies typically used in conventional medicine to treat acute low back pain are largely useless and possibly harmful, and that only one in a hundred people with low back pain benefit from surgery.[23]

Studies of Patient Satisfaction

From the consumer's point of view, studies of patient satisfaction are perhaps as important as studies of efficacy. One study compared the satisfaction levels of patients receiving allopathic care for low back pain with that of patients receiving chiropractic care. The latter group were found to have satisfaction levels three times as high as the former.[24]

Several other studies that have compared patient satisfaction with low back treatment by nurses, physical therapists, and chiropractors have also found the least satisfaction with medical doctors.[25,26,27,28]

Harvey

Harvey, a fifty-year-old overweight man, sought help for acute low back pain. He had developed symptoms of stenosis, meaning that his legs would become achy, tired, and painful when walking. He would pitch forward to get the weight off his back and legs.

He also had foot drop, which means he was not able to walk on his heels across a room nor could he walk on his toes. This indicates a serious compromise of the nerve impulses to the musculature of the legs and is one of the primary indications for discectomy, a form of spinal surgery that involves removal of a disc. Harvey also had a compromised achilles tendon reflex, which is another criterion commonly used in recommending surgery.

He was treated four times over an eleven-day period, at the end of which the foot drop was gone. Treatment included manual spinal manipulation and some intermittent motorized traction. He was also being treated with exercise therapy. The four treatments were twenty to thirty minutes and cost $50 each.

Cost-Effectiveness

Other research has compared the relative costs of chiropractic and medical care. A study of an insurance claims database of 1.1 million persons indicated that chiropractic users tend to have substantially lower total health care costs. Such patients were found to have a lower overall rate of inpatient utilization and they were also found to have lower total outpatient costs, even with the inclusion of the costs of chiropractic care. Hence these findings suggest that chiropractic helps reduce the utilization of both physician and hospital care.[29,30]

Another study examining workers' compensation in Utah compared the costs of medical claims and chiropractic claims for patients with identical diagnoses. Total compensation paid per case for all cases combined was significantly higher for those receiving medical treatment.[31]

STRENGTHS AND LIMITATIONS

The greatest strength of chiropractic is in treatment of neuromusculoskeletal conditions such as sprain- or strain-type injuries of the back and adjacent structures. According to Pammer, "Our strongest suit is low back conditions (as evidenced in the studies reported above). From there we go up into neck, head, and arm problems, especially migraine headaches, tension headaches, stiff necks, and torticollis. Our next strongest area would be extraspinal conditions such as problems in the knees, wrists, elbows, ankles, and other joints."

For low back pain, research has helped make it possible to predict fairly reliably which individuals will benefit. For conditions with more vague complaints or with visceral manifestation like gastritis, asthma, or allergies, the predictability of benefit is lower, although there is much anecdotal evidence that these conditions too can benefit.

Chiropractors do not treat fractures, perform major surgery, or prescribe medication. Clear limitations are in emergency medicine (trauma care), rapidly deteriorating conditions, acute infections, life-threatening diseases, or conditions that require invasive procedures.

All chiropractors are trained in obstetrics and gynecology. While they are capable of delivering babies, most states limit this. Rural states tend to allow a wider latitude of practice. In Washington they are allowed to perform minor surgery, though

Robert

Robert was a twenty-seven-year-old jewelry student. One day while moving some heavy furniture he twisted his back and over the next two weeks the pain became more intense. He went to see his physician, who referred him to an orthopedist who promptly ordered a myelogram (a procedure that was commonly used before the development of the MRI). He was found to have a herniated disc and the recommendation was surgery.

The surgical prognosis was described as "iffy" but it was considered his best option. The recommended procedure was a laminectomy fusion, which is the complete removal of the lamina (the posterior element of the spine) and deflection of the spinal cord. The fusion would take place by scraping bone fragments from the pelvis and patching them across the opening created by the surgical incision at the back of the spine.

While Robert agonized over the decision, obviously in a great deal of discomfort, a friend insisted on taking him to see the friend's chiropractor. Robert agreed, though he had never heard of chiropractic.

Upon his first visit, the chiropractor said, "You may have a herniated disc, but I think you have a problem in your pelvis and sacrum and that's what is giving you this trouble. Let's see if I can fix it and then we'll see if you need surgery."

After the spinal adjustment, Robert got off the table and was standing up straight with no more back pain. He was charged $7 for the visit (this was 1972). The chiropractor told him to return if he had any more trouble.

Some weeks later Robert banged his head on a door. The following day he had a severe headache and returned to the same chiropractor, who adjusted the cervical vertebra in his neck. Shortly thereafter the headache was gone.

As a result of this series of events, he decided to become a chiropractor. Robert Dubin, D.C., now practices in Petaluma, California. Twenty-two years have passed with no symptoms related to his herniated disc.

very few do. In some other states they are allowed to do minor surgery after taking an elective course, but this is rare.

Can many chiropractic adjustments over a long period of time weaken the spine? There is no scientific evidence of this. According to Meeker, "This speculation usually comes from people who don't really understand what chiropractic adjustments are all about. If you understand the nature of the forces that we use and you understand how the spine, ligaments, and joints behave over time, then it's really hard to see how this could actually happen."

THE PRACTITIONER-PATIENT RELATIONSHIP

As with other hands-on approaches to healing, the sense of empathy and rapport between practitioner and patient is a key to the professional relationship. Chiropractic care requires active verbal communication. The ongoing feedback from the patient during the course of a procedure often plays a key role in the process and there needs to be free communication for the work to be effective.

Many people grow very fond of their chiropractors because this unique combination of communication, empathy, and hands-on care fosters a sense of intimacy. Being handled gently and with confidence is a major reason for the wide popularity of this tradition. Another reason is the time many practitioners take to express a personal interest in the patient's lifestyle and its impact on their health.

EVALUATING PERSONAL RESULTS

Evaluation of results is a combination of the patient's subjective feedback along with the practitioner's objective findings, but patient self-report remains the most important indication of outcome. Practitioners also consider such measures as range of motion (ability to bend and touch the toes, bend backward and forward), change in various reflexes, changes in muscle tone or strength, heel tension, leg length, and changes in various structures or tissues they can feel through palpation. All of these may be recorded in progress notes.

Historically chiropractors have used X rays to show change, but these are on the decline because their reliability has been questioned.

There is an emerging trend toward more systematic measurement of outcomes by using more questionnaires or scales to assess progress over time. The chiropractic colleges have also begun to emphasize the use of such scales in regular office practice and this trend is propelled in part at least by health care reform and its quest for objective outcomes.

RELATIONSHIP TO OTHER FORMS OF MEDICINE

Until the antitrust suit against the American Medical Association was settled in 1987, relations between chiropractic and allopathy were quite strained. The AMA had an ethical precept for its members stating that to refer to or accept a referral from a chiropractor could lead to expulsion.

Since those days there has been steady improvement. Today almost all chiropractors have reciprocal referral relationships with M.D.s. Many interdisciplinary group practices include chiropractors and many hospitals have them on staff. While there are still some old-guard allopaths who continue to shun chiropractic, they are gradually disappearing.

Louise

Louise, thirty, had been suffering from acute sinusitis for three months. She had had antibiotics and, based on her X rays, surgery had been recommended. The procedure would involve cutting a hole behind her upper lip to insert a probe into her sinuses to evacuate them.

She decided to consult a chiropractor who happened to use craniosacral manipulation in his practice. This form of therapy has a specific protocol for sinusitis that works on the bone structures, muscles, and nerve structures that enervate and inhibit the sinus activity.

The practitioner wears a rubber glove and works inside the mouth. After two half-hour sessions Louise reported significant improvement and was breathing through her nose. Two weeks later she had a follow-up appointment with her surgeon, who took another X ray. He told her he was astounded at how improved her sinuses were because he would not expect to see such improvement even three months after surgery.

According to Robert Dubin, D.C., "I opened up the drains, the fluid poured out, and she was fine." He explains that the head is, in a sense, plumbed with a network of hoses and drains. "The sutures that separate the cranial plates are made up of articular tissue and proper alignment is necessary for proper drainage. I manipulated the sutures to reestablish normal alignment."

Chiropractic lends itself well to integration with other medical traditions as evidenced by the growing number of mixers who integrate nutritional therapy, homeopathy, and other natural therapies into their practice. It can be used as complementary therapy with any other tradition.

Part of chiropractic education includes training in the boundaries of chiropractic care and when to refer to allopathy. Sometimes allopathic drugs for pain control are required in conjunction with spinal manipulation, in which case a collaborative relationship with an allopath is helpful.

Chiropractors pride themselves on their efforts to help people avoid surgery if at all possible. However, there are cases that are clearly at a stage where they require more aggressive intervention. They may also refer for evaluation of particularly ambiguous cases.

COSTS

The initial visit takes forty-five to sixty minutes, with a case history, examination, and diagnostic tests, and may cost from $50 to $100 depending on the part of the country. A few practitioners give a free initial consultation for the purpose of meeting and interviewing the practitioner. Costs are generally lower in rural areas.

The cost of subsequent treatments may range from $20 to $50 for a ten to twenty-five minute visit. Approximately three-quarters of insurance companies (including Medicare) recognize and pay for chiropractic care and it is covered in all state workers' compensation acts.

Most treatment involves a series of visits. A typical range would be between three and fifteen visits, depending on the severity and chronicity of the problem. Spinal conditions are 85 percent of what chiropractors treat and Meeker estimates that with uncomplicated, biomechanical low back conditions, substantial improvement should generally be expected within twelve visits. If such improvement does not occur, then more testing, referral to a chiropractic orthopedist or radiologist, or an MRI may be indicated.

When there is disc involvement such as bulged or protruding (not herniated) disc, then the time frame may be longer. However, within twelve visits there should still be substantial change.

CHOOSING A PRACTITIONER

Licensing and Specialty Boards

Chiropractors are licensed in every state. In addition to graduating from an accredited college of chiropractic, they must also pass an examination with the National Board of Chiropractic Examiners. This is a two-part exam comparable to that of medical doctors. After completing this, they then take their individual state board exam. Finally, most states require a certain number of continuing education hours each year.

While there are several kinds of specialization available, as noted earlier, the vast majority of chiropractors operate without them. In reality, the various specializations are not widely available except perhaps in the larger urban areas. They include:

Diplomate of the American Chiropractic Board of Radiology (D.A.C.B.R.). These specialists often serve to provide second opinions on radiological questions to other chiropractors.

Diplomate of the American Chiropractic Board of Orthopedics (D.A.C.B.O.). The orthopedists specialize in sprain and strain injuries and may consult on the more complicated cases involving general chiropractic practice.

Chiropractic Council on Sports Injuries (C.C.S.I.). These are specifically trained in injuries related to on-field sports. This is a certification status, not a diplomate.

Diplomate of the American Chiropractic Board of Nutrition

Horace

Horace, forty, received a head injury from an encounter with a 150-pound door. His treatment had included muscle relaxants, pain medication, and rest for a month, but he was still in pain with a constant headache.

His initial chiropractic consultation included craniosacral manipulation and his headache disappeared while he was on the table. His cervical spine had also been damaged, so after the cranial work he was treated with manipulation and stretching of the cervical spine.

This case required extensive treatment, with thirty sessions over a period of four months. The sessions consisted of a combination of craniosacral manipulation, spinal adjustments, strengthening exercises, massage, ultrasound, and electrical stimulation to the muscles along the spine. At four months he was able to return to work pain-free.

(D.A.C.B.N.). These deal with the specialization of incorporating nutritional therapies into health care.

Diplomate of the American Chiropractic Board of Internists (D.A.C.B.I.). They are specialists in use of laboratory tests and other diagnostic procedures dealing with the interface of chiropractic and internal medicine.

Diplomate of the American Chiropractic Board of Neurologists (D.A.C.B.N.). These are chiropractors who have advanced training in neurological conditions and diseases of the nervous system.

Straight or Mixer?

A key question is whether you wish to see a practitioner who concentrates only on spinal manipulation or integrates other approaches to health. This is more important if you are going to include chiropractic in your long-term health maintenance plans and less important if you are in a crisis with severe back pain. In the latter case, you probably want relief from pain as quickly as possible and this demands chiropractic's unique strength, the variety of spinal manipulations available regardless of the practitioner's other interests.

If you choose to work with a mixer, then you can inquire about the extent of their training in the other modalities they offer. For instance, they may have advanced training or certification in homeopathy, acupuncture, nutritional therapies, a form of bodywork, or Ayurveda.

Organizations

There are over 48,000 chiropractors, but there is no single organization that has a majority of membership. Many practitioners do not belong to any and none is required for licensure. The organizations that most people are likely to hear about are as follows:

International Chiropractic Association, founded by B. J. Palmer, is the oldest association. It promotes the subluxation-based approach. A voluntary membership organization, it provides a variety of educational materials for the general public to advance the profession and also publishes *The ICA Review,* a bimonthly journal. Address: 1110 N. Glebe Rd., Suite 1000, Arlington, VA 22201, phone (800) 423–4690.

American Chiropractic Association, the association with the largest membership, publishes the *Journal of the American Chiropractic Association* and promotes ethical and professional

263

Joline

Joline, eighteen, had just finished cosmetology school and had been experiencing disabling knee pain during and after work. Her physician told her she had osteochondrosis, also known as Osgood/Schlatter's disease. She was prescribed anti-inflammatory drugs but had difficulty with an upset stomach as a side effect.

Her chiropractor determined she had some pelvic instability. He adjusted her full spine, her knees, ankles, and feet. She reported immediate improvement and now is working all day without pain.

standards, public education, research, and legislative leadership for the profession. Each state also has a state chapter. Address: 1701 Clarendon Blvd., Arlington, VA 22209, phone (703) 276–8800.

World Chiropractic Alliance is another voluntary membership organization for public education and advocacy of the profession. It publishes two periodicals, *True Health* and *The Chiropractic Journal*. Address: 2950 N. Dobson Rd., Suite 1, Chandler, AZ 85224, phone (800) 347–1011.

Association for Network Chiropractic requires as training for membership a series of four weekend seminars in Network Chiropractic. A directory of practitioners (just over five hundred nationwide) is available. Address: 444 North Main St., Longmont, CO 80501, phone (303) 678–8101.

Conclusion

The basic criterion in choosing a practitioner is an active license. Beyond this, useful questions are whether they are a straight or mixer, to whom they refer when a physician referral is necessary, and whether they insist on costly X rays (since there is little scientific support for their extensive use, particularly for most cases of low back pain).

You may also want to get an estimate of how many sessions the practitioner feels are needed for your treatment since such estimates may vary widely. This will give you an idea of their approach in terms of minimizing unnecessary treatment. Their willingness to take time to explain how they work with your condition is also a good sign.

As with any health care tradition, you need to determine whether you feel personally comfortable in the practitioner's presence and whether they elicit a sense of trust within you. Personal word-of-mouth recommendations are always a good idea.

CHAPTER 9

MASSAGE THERAPY AND BODYWORK: HEALING THROUGH TOUCH

"The physician must be experienced in many things, but most assuredly in rubbing."

—HIPPOCRATES

Hands-on manipulation for healing is probably older than any other healing tradition. The oldest written records of massage go back three thousand years to China, but of course it is much older than that. Touch and the laying on of hands are human tendencies that seem to be in our genetic makeup.

Physicians and healers of all forms and from all cultures have used hands-on manipulation throughout history as an integral part of health care practice. In the former Soviet countries, Germany, Japan, and China, massage has continued uninterrupted as massage therapists today work alongside doctors as part of the health care team.

In modern Germany massage therapy is covered by national health insurance. In China it is fully integrated into the health care system, where the hospitals have massage wards. In

266

one Shanghai hospital the massage department covers two floors.

In this country, the medical use of massage began to diminish in the early part of this century with the evolution of pharmaceutical, surgical, and technological medicine. It reached a nadir in the 1930s, 40s, and 50s because it was considered too time-intensive for the modern physician. Massage therapy duties were gradually handed over to aides, who eventually became the physical therapists of the modern era.

The professionalization of massage therapy in the United States began in 1943 when the graduating class of the College of Swedish Massage in Chicago decided to band together and form an association with twenty-nine charter members. What they created was destined to become the American Massage Therapy Association (AMTA).

In the 1960s, while modern medicine continued its march toward higher technology and drugs and away from physician contact with patients, such concepts as holistic health, self-improvement, and optimal health experienced a rebirth. The 1970s brought even greater interest in health promotion and a new openness to massage.

This was followed by explosive growth in the varieties of massage and bodywork available, and today there are now over eighty different varieties. The term "bodywork" evolved as a generic term for referring to this broadening field. It is now loosely used to incorporate massage and other forms of manipulation.

In the survey of alternative medicine that was published in *The New England Journal of Medicine* in January 1993,[1] massage therapy ranked third among the most frequently used forms of alternative health care. According to Elliot Greene, president of the AMTA, there are now an estimated fifty thousand massage therapists of various kinds in the United States, and the AMTA may be the fastest-growing organization of health care providers in the country. At this writing it has over eighteen thousand members and its rolls have more than doubled in the last three years.

Education

There are myriad programs of education and training for the many different forms of massage and bodywork. For the massage therapy field, the AMTA has been successful in establishing standards that are incorporated in many state licensing laws. Fifty-eight training programs are currently accredited or approved by the AMTA-affiliated Commission on Massage Training Accreditation/Approval, which requires at least five hundred hours of classroom instruction. The curriculum includes three hundred hours of massage theory and technique, one hundred hours of anatomy and physiology, and one hundred hours of additional required courses including first aid and cardiopulmonary resuscitation (CPR). There are of course many other training programs that do not meet all of these standards.

Training in other forms of bodywork is much less uniform and there are no licensing laws for bodywork methods as such. Many bodyworkers are also massage therapists, but this is not required for most bodywork traditions. The various associations described later in this chapter all have their own unique standards for training.

KEY PRINCIPLES

While there are a wide variety of forms of massage therapy and bodywork, all with their own theoretical or philosophical perspectives, there are certain basic principles they all tend to hold in common.

Circulation of Blood. Perhaps the most basic principle in this field is that improved blood circulation is beneficial for virtually all health conditions. Tension in the muscles and other soft tissues can impair circulation, resulting in a deficient supply of nutrients and inadequate removal of wastes or toxins from the

Elena

Elena, a twenty-five-year-old graduate student, had suffered a back injury as a result of a cheerleading accident
when she was fifteen. She was at the bottom of a pyra-
mid on all fours when someone fell on her back from
ten feet in the air and she received a severe strain and
sprain to the thoracic vertebra and lower back. For ten
years she had struggled with chronic pain in the soft
tissue throughout the area. She had fatigue as a result
of the pain and a loss of range of movement in her
back.

She had received chiropractic, acupuncture, pharmaceutical, and physical therapy but had made only moderate progress. At first she was diagnosed with fibrositis.
Later, with no positive findings by X ray, the suspicion
was that she had a psychological disorder.

Elena's mother initiated contact with a massage therapist. He noted immediately that the third and fourth
thoracic vertebra were depressed and began a regimen
of a deep tissue technique called cross-fiber work on
the affected areas of her back. She was seen four times
over a month, each week reporting steady improvement.

Elliot Greene describes the process as one of breaking
up the scarring that had occurred in her muscles and
connective tissue or fascia between the muscles, vertebra, and ribs, all of which had become stuck together.
Blood flow through the area was restored and the depression that had been palpable in her spine gradually
began to diminish. The full range of motion of the spine
returned.

tissues of the body. This in turn can lead to illness, structural and functional problems, or slower healing. Recognition of the importance of blood circulation is implicit in all forms of massage and bodywork.

Movement of Lymphatic Fluid. The lymph system is almost as extensive as that of the blood. The circulation of lymphatic fluid plays a key role in ridding the body of wastes, toxins, and pathogens. The lymph system also benefits from massage, particularly in conditions where lymphatic flow is impaired by injury or surgery (e.g., in postmastectomy women).

Release of Toxins. Chronic tension or trauma to the soft tissues of the body can result in the buildup of toxic by-products of normal metabolism. Hands-on techniques help move the toxins through the body's normal pathways of release and elimination.

Release of Tension. Chronic muscular tension as a result of high-stress lifestyles, trauma, or injury can accumulate and impair the body's structure and function. Psychological well-being is also affected. Release of tension allows greater relaxation, which has important physiological and psychological benefits.

Structure and Function Are Interdependent. The musculoskeletal structure of the body affects function and function affects structure. Both can be adversely altered by stress or trauma. Massage therapy and bodywork can help restore healthy structure and function, thereby allowing better circulation, greater ease of movement, wider range of movement, more flexibility, and the release of chronic patterns of tension.

Enhancement of All Bodily Systems. All bodily systems are affected by better circulation and more harmonious functioning of the soft tissue and musculature. Internal organ systems as well as the nervous system, the immune system, and other systems can benefit. There can be an overall improvement in the quality of life and physical health.

Mind/Body Integration. Mind and body have a reciprocal relationship. Soma (body) affects psyche (mind) and vice versa. Hence there can be somatopsychic effects, in which the conditions of the body affect the mind and emotions, and there can be psychosomatic effects, in which psychological or emotional conditions affect the body. Change in one domain may cause change in the other. A habit or fixed pattern in one may also impede change in the other and require special attention. Often psychotherapy and massage or bodywork complement each other.

Reduction of Stress. Stress is increasingly believed to induce illness, and perhaps 80 to 90 percent of all disease is stress-induced. Massage therapy is an effective nondrug method for reducing stress and promoting relaxation.

Energy. Many modalities in this tradition work with the flow of energy through the body as a means to promote healing. Energy can be directed or encouraged to move through and around the body in such ways as to have impact on the physical structure and function of the body as well as on emotional well-being. This work may involve hands-on contact or may be done with no contact with the physical body.

According to Joanna Chieppa, R.M.T., a faculty member at Heartwood Institute in Garberville, California, and an energy healing practitioner in Sonoma County, "It is important for people to develop an awareness that the flow of energy in and around the body is just as important to well-being as the flow of blood, the flow of breath, the flow of cerebral spinal fluid— that it is essential for the health of body, mind, and spirit."[2]

VARIETIES AND TECHNIQUES

For this chapter, the sections on varieties and techniques are combined. As stated earlier, there are over eighty different types of massage therapy and bodywork. Many are variations on each other, often developed by a practitioner who is trained in one particular approach and then goes on to develop his or her own variety, with its own new "brand name."

Most varieties can be broken down into the following five broad categories:

Traditional European Massage
Contemporary Western Massage
Structural/Functional/Movement Integration
Oriental Methods
Energetic Methods (Nonoriental)

The majority of activity in this field is oriented toward the traditional European and contemporary Western forms of massage simply because there are such large numbers of practitioners of these methods.

Traditional European Massage

Traditional European massage includes methods based on conventional Western concepts of anatomy and physiology and soft tissue manipulation. There are five basic kinds of soft tissue manipulation techniques: effleurage (long flowing or gliding strokes, usually toward the heart, tracing the outer contours of the body), petrissage (strokes that lift, roll, or knead the tissue), friction (circular strokes), vibration, and tapotement (percussion or tapping).

Traditional European massage was brought to the United States by two doctors from New York who were brothers— Charles and George Taylor—who studied in Sweden and introduced Americans to Swedish techniques in the 1850s. After the Civil War, the first Swedish clinics opened in Boston and Washington, the latter frequented by U. S. Grant.

Swedish Massage. Swedish massage is by far the most predominant example of traditional European massage and it is the most commonly used method in the United States. It was developed by Per Henrik Ling in Sweden in the 1830s and uses a system of long gliding strokes, kneading, and friction techniques on the more superficial layers of muscles. It usually goes in the direction of blood flow toward the heart because there is an emphasis on stimulating the circulation of the blood through the soft tissues of the body. Swedish can be a relatively vigorous form of massage, sometimes with a great deal of joint movement included.

Oil is usually used, which facilitates the stroking and kneading of the body, thereby stimulating metabolism and circulation. Its active and passive movements of the joints promote general relaxation, improve circulation and range of motion, and relieve muscle tension. Swedish massage is often given as a complete, full body technique, though sometimes only a part of the body is worked on.

Contemporary Western Massage

This includes methods based primarily on modern Western concepts of human function, anatomy, and physiology, using a wide variety of manipulative techniques. These may include broad applications for personal growth, emotional release, and balance of mind-body-spirit in addition to traditional applications. These approaches go beyond the original framework or intention of Swedish massage. They include Esalen or Swedish/Esalen, neuromuscular massage, deep tissue massage, sports massage, and manual lymph drainage. Most of these are American techniques developed from the late 1960s onward, though the latter was developed in the 1920s.

Esalen and Swedish/Esalen. Esalen massage is a modern variation that was developed at the famous growth center, Esalen Institute in Big Sur, California. Its focus is not so much on relieving muscle tension or increasing circulation as it is on creating deeper states of relaxation, beneficial states of consciousness, and general well-being. Whereas Swedish is more brisk and focuses on the body, Esalen is more slow, rhythmic, and hypnotic and focuses on the mind/body as a whole.

Esalen massage is not widely taught as a pure form. Rather, a marriage of sorts has been formed by the integration of Swedish and Esalen as a way of incorporating the strengths of each. Many massage therapists describe their method as Swedish/Esalen, and this hybrid is commonly taught in massage schools.

Neuromuscular Massage. This is a form of deep massage that applies concentrated finger pressure specifically to individual muscles. This is a very detailed approach, used to increase blood flow and to release trigger points, intense knots of muscle tension that refer pain to other parts of the body (they become trigger points when they seem to trigger a pain pattern). This form of massage helps to break the cycle of spasm and pain and is often used in pain control. Trigger point massage and myotherapy are varieties of neuromuscular massage.

Deep Tissue Massage. This approach is used to release chronic patterns of muscular tension using slow strokes, direct pressure, or friction. Often the movements are directed across the grain of the muscles (cross-fiber) using the fingers, thumbs, or elbows. This is applied with greater pressure and at deeper layers of the muscle than Swedish massage and that is why it is called deep tissue.

It is also more specific. For example, in the case of someone with a sore shoulder, the practitioner may focus on the trapezius and the rhomboid underneath, trying to work in all the layers of muscle that might be involved. Deep tissue massage lends itself to being more focused on a problem area.

Sports Massage. This uses techniques similar to Swedish and deep tissue but more specifically adapted to deal with the needs of athletes and the effects of athletic performance on the body.

Frederick

Frederick, a forty-eight-year-old attorney, was chopping wood in his garden when he pulled a muscle on his right shoulder blade. He had always been very active but was now unable to play tennis because his arm and shoulder would cramp up. He was even unable to sit down and write a letter because of the cramping.

His physician gave him steroid injections and sent him to physical therapy for two months, which helped eliminate some but not all of the pain. The physical therapy included ultrasound and electrical stimulation.

The massage therapist found him to have extreme spasms and tension of the muscles on the back of the shoulder blade, some of which were like rock. The therapist initiated very precisely focused, deep transverse friction cross-fiber work, as much as possible right on the places where the muscles had been damaged. Frederick was seen weekly for about a year, after which he now has full use of his shoulder and arm and can do gardening work without pain.

As Elliot Greene explains, the problem with severe spasm is that it cuts off its own circulation and becomes a self-reinforcing syndrome. This is another case of opening up the flow of blood and lymph through the area, releasing adhesions, and using deep transverse friction to encourage the unhealed part of the muscle to heal.

Sports massage is used before or after events, as part of an athlete's training regimen, and to promote healing from injuries.

Manual Lymph Drainage Massage. This approach improves the flow of lymph using light rhythmic strokes. It is used primarily in conditions characterized by poor lymph flow, such as edema.

Structural/Functional/Movement Integration

These approaches organize and integrate the body in relationship to gravity through manipulating the soft tissues, and/or through correcting inappropriate patterns of movement. These are methods that bring about more balanced use of the body and nervous system, creating greater integration and more ease of movement.

This category of approaches is interesting in that some do not even involve the practitioner touching the client. There is no clear line of demarcation between where the bodywork therapies end and the movement therapies begin. Furthermore, many practitioners use multiple techniques that integrate massage, deeper tissue work, and movement all in the same session with a client.

These approaches work on the body structure and how it moves. The most common approaches include Rolfing, Hellerwork, the Rosen Method, the Trager approach, the Feldenkrais Method, the Alexander Technique, and Ortho-Bionomy.

Rolfing. Rolfing is the most established method in this category. There are over eight hundred Rolfers practicing in twenty-seven countries, with about seven hundred in the United States.

Rolfing is a trademarked approach within the generic field of structural integration. It was developed by Ida Rolf, Ph.D., a biophysicist who earned her doctorate in the 1920s. She began doing her form of bodywork in the 1940s and 50s. Her clientele included Georgia O'Keeffe and Buckminster Fuller and she worked with other pioneers in the bodywork field. In the 1960s she began teaching at Esalen Institute. She formed the Rolf Institute of Structural Integration in Boulder, Colorado, in 1972.

Rolfing involves a form of deep tissue work for reordering the body so as to bring its major segments—head, shoulder, thorax, pelvis, and legs—into a finer vertical alignment. The technique loosens or releases adhesions in the fascia, the flexible tissue that envelops our muscles and muscle groups. The fascia is supposed to move easily and allow easy articulation or movement of muscles or muscle groups past each other. However, trauma such as injury or chronic stress can cause stuck points or adhesions, in which the fascia is in a sense frozen, not allowing full freedom of movement.

The Rolfer works to restore this freedom of movement, resulting in a more balanced, vertical alignment of the body and often a lengthening or expansion of the body's trunk. Rolfing usually takes place over a series of ten organized sessions dealing with different areas of the body.

Hellerwork. This approach was founded by Joseph Heller in 1979. A former Rolfer, Heller developed a method that, along with structural reintegration, incorporates a movement reeducation process with exercises that teach stress-free methods for performing everyday movements such as standing, walking, bending, sitting, and reaching. (Since he left the Rolf Institute, Rolfing has also incorporated movement in its work.) Heller's approach often includes video feedback to show clients how they move.

Hellerwork takes place in a series of eleven sessions. Each session includes about an hour of bodywork and a half hour of movement education. There are over 160 certified Hellerwork practitioners in twenty-three states and seven foreign countries.

Rosen Method. Marion Rosen began her career in the 1930s and is still actively teaching her technique today. She founded her training program in 1972. The Rosen Method sees the body's tensions as indications of unexpressed feelings or other repressed or suppressed aspects of the self. The result of such holding patterns, which may be very subtle, can be lifelong patterns of tension or organic malfunction.

The Rosen Method uses gentle, nonintrusive touch and verbal

exchange between practitioner and client to help draw the client's attention to areas of holding. This serves to help the client become fully aware of how the patterns of tension are associated with emotional or unconscious material. This awareness itself is the key that allows the tension or holding patterns to be released. Often the tightness softens and the area that was being held begins to move easily with the breath.

In the words of Marion Rosen, "This work is about transformation, from the person we think we are to the person we really are."

Trager. The Trager approach is a system of movement reeducation or psychophysical integration developed by Milton Trager, M.D. It uses gentle, noninvasive movements to help release deep-seated physical and mental patterns and in turn allow deeper relaxation, increased physical mobility, and better mental clarity.

A session is one to one and a half hours. The practitioner moves the client's trunk and limbs in a gentle, rhythmic way so that the person experiences new sensations of freedom of movement. The practitioner's concern is fostering a sense of freedom and lightness.

After the hands-on portion of the session, the client is given instruction in the use of Mentastics, a system of movement sequences developed by Trager for the purpose of re-creating and enhancing the sense of lightness and ease of movement initiated on the table. The benefits of the Trager approach are cumulative, though there is no set series of sessions.

Feldenkrais Method. This approach was developed by Moshe Feldenkrais, a Russian-born Israeli educator. It uses physical movement to focus learning on the juncture of thought and action. It is known for its ability to improve posture and flexibility and alleviate muscular tension and pain.

It works with the nervous system's capacity for change and learning new patterns for moving, feeling, and thinking. The method involves two applications: Awareness Through Movement (ATM) and Functional Integration (FI). ATM consists

John

John was a veteran of the Vietnam War who was still suffering from a war injury many years later. He had been dropped from a helicopter into a battle from six or seven feet up and landed on his shoulder with all of his weight. The medics gave him some injections and sent him back out into the field, so he never received any real therapy. Since his return home the injury had become chronic over many years. He had limited range of motion in his arm and was unable to perform in sports, which had been his hobby.

His massage therapist determined that there was deep damage to the deltoid muscle, which had been crushed, and the scarring of the muscle had adhered to the bone and become hardened. In fact he had an area about the size of a quarter deep in the muscle that felt like bone. After deep tissue work the area began to come alive again and over time he was able to enjoy sports again.

Elliot Greene explains, "Sometimes when you get a deep bruise to a muscle it actually calcifies. Also, when scar tissue does not heal well the fibers of the scar can grow in a matted way that impairs movement of muscle tissue—the scar tissue may cross the muscle fibers and restrict them.

"Then, through the adhesions that are formed around the scar, these tissues become stuck to adjacent tissues. In John's case they became stuck to the periosteum, the skin that covers the bone. This is why when he would try to move this muscle, there would be a stabbing pain.

"This particular case took a lot of strength to break up the adhesions. With deep tissue therapy, after the scar begins to soften, the fibers begin to move more parallel to the muscle fibers, thus being less resistant to movement of the muscle tissue. This is 'the stretch hypertrophy law.' Also, the opening up of circulation of lymph and blood helped unfreeze the area."

of verbally directed, pleasurable, and effortless exercise lessons involving highly sophisticated movement sequences. FI is a one-on-one process that involves the use of specific skilled touch and passive movement. It is known for its ability to address serious muscular and neurological problems and improve human functioning.

The Alexander Technique. This is an approach to psychophysical reeducation. It was developed by the Australian actor F. M. Alexander and works with unconscious patterns of thinking and the resultant movements or postures that become set in the musculature. Such patterns can be made conscious so the student can then become aware of how he/she moves and can make the choice to change patterns, allowing more balance, grace, and ease of movement, thereby reducing and eliminating chronic tension or distortion in the musculoskeletal system. The relationships among the head, neck, and back are of particular importance.

The Alexander Technique is taught in private half-hour to hour lessons. The teacher works with the student to observe and change mind/body habits that interfere with optimal functioning. The teacher uses both verbal and hands-on guidance to help the student experience new ways of moving and embodying him- or herself. It is not a fixed series of treatments or exercises, but often a series of several lessons is recommended. Training to become a teacher takes three years (sixteen hundred hours).

Ortho-Bionomy. Ortho-Bionomy was developed in the 1970s by the bodyworker Arthur Lincoln Pauls. This approach uses gentle, relaxing movements and postures to help the body release tensions and muscular holding patterns. No force or pressure from the practitioner is used. Its goal is a restoration of structural alignment and balance.

Oriental Methods

Oriental methods are based on the principles of Chinese medicine and the flow of energy or *chi* through the meridians. The geography of the acupuncture meridians is relied upon to determine points of applying the techniques and the ultimate goal is restoration of harmony or balance in the flow of *chi*. These forms may also be used in concert with herbs and acupuncture.

Pressure is applied by finger or thumb tips to predetermined points rather than by the sweeping broad strokes of Western-style massage. Strong pressure or very light pressure may be applied. There are over a dozen varieties of oriental massage and bodywork therapy, but the most common forms in this country are acupressure, shiatsu, Jin Shin Jyutsu, and Jin Shin Do® Bodymind Acupressure™.

Acupressure and Shiatsu. These are similar varieties of finger pressure massage. They are both based on applying pressure to a pattern of specific points that correspond with the acupuncture points. Pressure is applied with the thumb, finger, and palm rather than needles.

The goal is the efficient and balanced flow of *chi* through the meridians. It is believed that where there is tension being held in the musculature, the flow of *chi* is impaired through those areas, which can lead to chronic problems not only in the musculature but in the associated organs. Stretching and movement are also sometimes used.

Acupressure is the more generic term used for this approach and shiatsu is the Japanese version.

Jin Shin Jyutsu. This approach comes from an ancient Japanese healing tradition that uses touch to restore the internal flow of energy through the body by releasing energetic blockages. A session lasts about an hour and the client is fully clothed, lying on a table. The practitioner uses pulse diagnosis to identify energy blocks and then gently holds or touches a specific combi-

281

nation of two of twenty-six acupuncture points to allow release of the blockage.

As it is practiced in the United States the holding uses less pressure than other forms of acupressure or shiatsu and there is no application of massagelike movements to specific points. Rather the touch is very light and works to balance the flow of energy.

Jin Shin Do® Bodymind Acupressure™. This approach was developed by California psychotherapist Iona Marsaa Tee-guarden. It applies stronger acupressure on the points and for a longer period of time than does Jin Shin Jyutsu. It focuses on the deep release of armoring (muscular tension of physical or emotional origins) through gentle yet deep finger pressure.

Jin Shin Do® incorporates Taoist breathing techniques, oriental acupuncture theory, Japanese finger pressure technique (sometimes holding points for as much as one to three minutes), and Reichian segmental theory (an understanding of how tensions in different parts of the body affect each other as well as particular feelings or emotions).

Energetic Methods (Nonoriental)

In a sense, all the oriental methods described above are also energetic methods in that they are working with energy according to principles of Chinese medicine and view the human being as an energy system. However, there are other energetic methods that are not based on Chinese principles. The most prominent of these are Therapeutic Touch, polarity therapy, and Reiki.

Therapeutic Touch. This method is unique in that it was born and reached its maturation within the context of conventional Western medicine. It was developed in the 1970s by Dolores

Krieger, Ph.D., R.N., a professor at New York University, and Dora Kunz, a natural healer. It is a contemporary interpretation of several ancient healing traditions.

It is based on the principle that the human energy field extends beyond the skin and the practitioner can use the hands as sensors to locate problems in it that correspond with problems in the physical body. Disease is seen as a condition of energy imbalance or blocked energy flow. Assessment is done by passing the hands over the body from head to toe at about two to four inches above the surface.

The practitioner then serves as a conduit for universal energy, consciously and actively transferring energy into the recipient. The hands are used to direct and focus the energy, sometimes in rhythmical, sweeping motions. The method is initially taught "off body," meaning the practitioner's hands do not touch the physical body, though later with experience some physical touch may take place.

Since it is not necessary to touch the physical body (what is being touched is the energy field or energy body), this method can be applied in situations where the patient may not be able to tolerate contact (e.g., in postsurgical patients or burn victims). Sessions last up to thirty minutes and can be done sitting or lying down fully clothed.

Therapeutic Touch is currently taught in over eighty universities and thirty countries and is practiced by twenty to thirty thousand health care professionals in the United States and around the world.

Polarity Therapy. This is a form of energy work that was developed by Randolph Stone, a chiropractor, osteopath, and naturopath in the mid-1920s. The practitioner uses subtle touch or holding on specific points to harmonize the flow of energy through the body and also to enhance the body's structural balance.

It is based on the principle that every cell has both negative and positive poles and the body is gently manipulated to enhance the energy flow. Emotional tension or physical pain are released

Joan

Joan was a thirty-two-year-old graduate student about to receive her Ph.D. in geology. She was also engaged but had a lot of anxieties about getting married. She sought massage therapy because of chronic headaches. Upon palpating her neck and upper shoulders, the practitioner found the muscles to be very knotty and hard. They had obviously been chronically tense for a long time.

During the course of several sessions Joan began to realize there was a relationship between the headaches, the tension she was holding in her musculature, and memories of having been physically abused as a child. The practitioner encouraged her to explore this with a psychotherapist.

She came back a year later for another series of four sessions. When the tense areas were encountered, she responded differently from before by telling the practitioner, "This really hurts," whereas in the past she had said nothing. The practitioner suggested she rephrase this by saying "I hurt," at which she began to sob as she never had before.

This was a very cleansing kind of release and through it Joan realized that in childhood she had adopted a pattern of numbing out to escape painful feelings. Through four sessions of massage she was able to release that long-held pattern and her fear and mistrust of her fiancé also ceased.

As Elliot Greene states, "It is very common that someone will come in for one reason, and then they will discover another whole dimension to the problem or to themselves that they want to explore."

as the flow of energy becomes more properly balanced. Polarity therapy is often given in a series of four sessions and may be accompanied by guidelines for diet and exercise.

Reiki. This is the Japanese word for "universal life force energy." It is an ancient approach in which the practitioner is a kind of healer in the sense that he or she serves as a conduit for healing energy coming from the universe.

The Reiki energy enters the practitioner through the top of the head and exits through the hands, being directed into the body or energy field of the recipient. Reiki is another very subtle form of healing and may be done through clothing and without any physical contact between practitioner and client.

While all the above energetic methods appear to operate on different principles than most other varieties of massage therapy and bodywork, they nonetheless have an important and growing role.

Other Approaches

Integrative Methods. There are other approaches and combinations of approaches that do not fit neatly into any of the above categories. Many massage therapists and bodyworkers use combinations of approaches that could be called integrative massage or integrative bodywork.

CranioSacral Therapy™. This approach was named in 1977 by John Upledger, D.O., and Ernest Retzlaff, Ph.D., to distinguish it from Sutherland's cranial osteopathy. According to Upledger, "CranioSacral Therapy is not osteopathy. Sutherland's approach was bone-oriented and you make bony corrections. This is soft tissue-oriented, fluid-oriented, membrane-oriented, and energy-oriented. It's much more subtle than any other kind of cranial work I know of."[3]

Palpation (touch by the practitioner) is used both to observe and treat dysfunctions in the craniosacral system, which includes the head, spinal column, and sacrum in one continuous membranous sheath. This system has its own pulse for circulating the cerebrospinal fluid (six to twelve cycles per minute) and the practitioner can feel the rate, amplitude, symmetry, and quality of the rhythm—somewhat analogous to pulse diagnosis in Ayurveda and Chinese medicine. Corrective pressure of only about five grams (the weight of a nickel) is applied to various areas to promote the reestablishment of a normal, symmetrical pattern of pulsation throughout the system. This in turn allows more efficient functioning of the entire nervous system throughout the body.

Upledger reports success in treating chronic pain, chronic brain dysfunctions when there is no structural problem involved, endogenous depression, migraines, learning disabilities, dyslexia, hyperkinesis, spasticity in cerebral palsy, strabismus (cross-eyes), Ménière's disease (vertigo), and many other conditions.

Reflexology. This approach involves the manual stimulation of reflex points on the ears, hands, and feet. Similar methods resembling shiatsu and acupressure have also been practiced in China for thousands of years. Thumb pressure is applied to specific points that correspond somatotopically to specific areas or organs of the body.

Reflexology was introduced to this country by William Fitzgerald, who termed it "zone therapy," in the early 1900s. One of the contemporary explanations for how it works is that compression by specific touch techniques affects a system of points and areas that are thought to "reflex" through neurological pathways to distant parts of the body. The pressure on these reflex points (also called "cuteneo-organ reflex points") is used to relieve stress and tension, to improve blood supply, to promote the unblocking of nerve impulses, and to help restore homeostasis or balance in the body.[4]

Zero Balancing. This is a painless, hands-on method of aligning body energy with body structure. It is done through clothes and involves the practitioner in using gentle pressure at key areas

286

of the skeleton in order to balance the energy body with the structural body.

The theory holds that each of us has an unseen energy body that exists like a glove surrounding the physical body. When injury or trauma occurs, healing of these two bodies does not necessarily occur simultaneously. "Balancing" refers to balancing the relationship between energy and structure. Zero Balancing seeks to bridge the gap between those methods that work with structure and those working with energy.

SCIENTIFIC SUPPORT

Prior to the advent of pharmaceutical medicine earlier in this century, references to massage therapy and research were not uncommon in the mainstream medical literature. There were over six hundred articles in various journals such as the *Journal of the American Medical Association, British Medical Journal,* and others from 1813 to 1939. A great deal of research was also conducted in Eastern Bloc countries and China. In this country after World War I, there was a precipitous decline in focus on this field as drugs and other allopathic interventions gained the foreground.

With the renewed interest in natural forms of treatment, research activity in massage and bodywork has again gained momentum. Studies have documented benefits for amputations, arthritis, cerebral palsy, cerebral vascular accident, fibrositis syndrome, menstrual cramps, paraplegia/quadriplegia, scoliosis, acute and chronic pain, acute and chronic inflammation, chronic lymphedema, nausea, muscle spasm, soft tissue dysfunctions, grand mal epileptic seizures, anxiety, depression, insomnia, and psychoemotional stress, which may aggravate significant mental illness. Following are a few examples of recent studies.

Massage in the Elderly. A controlled study showed massage therapy produced relaxation in eighteen elderly subjects. This

OAM-Funded Studies

When the Office of Alternative Medicine at NIH invited applications for its initial wave of research grants, eighty-five of the 450 applications were for massage-related studies, the largest number of any modality. Of the first thirty grants awarded, the following four dealt with massage therapy:

Thomas Burk, Ph.D., of the Morse Physical Health Research Center in Toledo, Ohio, was awarded a grant to study whether immune functioning could be improved in AIDS patients when massage therapy was used in combination with antiviral drugs.

Denise Matt Tope, Ph.D., of Dartmouth College in Hanover, New Hampshire, was awarded funds to study whether massage therapy can reduce anxiety and depression in bone marrow transplant patients.

Douglas DeGood, Ph.D., at the University of Virginia was funded to study the degree to which massage therapy can reduce anxiety and the need for follow-up care in women undergoing surgery for uterine cancer.

Frank Scafidi, Ph.D., at the University of Miami's Touch Research Institute is studying the effects of daily massage on growth, cognitive development, and immune function in premature infants born to HIV-infected mothers.

A fifth study involves Therapeutic Touch. Melodie Olson of the Medical University of South Carolina in Charleston is using a controlled experiment to examine the effects of Therapeutic Touch on the immune functioning of highly stressed students preparing for professional board exams. Positive findings would have implications for other highly stressed populations including cancer and AIDS patients.

study demonstrated physiological signs of relaxation in terms of decreased blood pressure and heart rate and increased skin temperature.[5]

Spinal Pain. A study of the combination of various types of massage in fifty-two patients with traumatically induced spinal pain led to significant reductions in acute and chronic pain and increased muscle flexibility and tone. This study also found massage to be extremely cost-effective in comparison with other pain therapies, with cost savings ranging from 15 to 50 percent.[6]

Pain Control. Massage has also been shown to stimulate the body's ability to control pain naturally. One study showed that massage stimulates the brain to produce endorphins, chemicals that control pain.[7]

Lymphedema. Lymph drainage massage has been found to be more effective than mechanized methods or diuretic drugs to control lymphedema (a form of swelling) caused by radical mastectomy. It can be expected that using massage to control lymphedema will significantly lower treatment costs. This is based on a study comparing massage with the use of sleevelike pressure cuffs often worn by women with lymphedema.[8]

Inflammatory Bowel Disease. A study found that massage therapy can have a powerful effect on psychoemotional distress in patients with chronic inflammatory bowel diseases such as ulcerative colitis and Crohn's disease. Stress can worsen the symptoms of these conditions, which can lead to great pain, bleeding, and hospitalization or death. Massage therapy was effective in reducing the frequency of episodes of pain and disability in these patients.[9]

Therapeutic Touch and Wound Healing. A controlled trial examined the effects of Therapeutic Touch on healing identical surgically inflicted minor wounds in the shoulders of forty-four male college students. Twenty-three received Therapeutic Touch treatments and twenty-one did not. Neither group was aware of the purpose of the experiment and those treated were not aware they were being treated. After eight days, the treated group's wounds had shrunk an average of 93.5 percent compared to 67.3 percent for those untreated. After sixteen days the figures were 99.3 percent and 90.9 percent.[10]

Reflexology and PMS. A controlled clinical study of thirty-eight women with premenstrual syndrome examined the effects of a thirty-minute reflexology treatment weekly for eight weeks. Those receiving the treatment were treated by ear, hand, and foot reflexology. Those in the control group were given placebo or sham reflexology. Based on a daily diary that monitored the severity of thirty-eight premenstrual symptoms, the treated group had a 46-percent reduction, which was a significantly greater reduction than the 19-percent reduction of the control group.

Unlike some of the hormone-altering drugs and antidepressant medications that are often used, the treatment produced no side effects. The researchers concluded that reflexology might work by softening adrenocortical reactivity to stress, which is known to exacerbate symptoms in PMS.[11]

Touch Research Institute, University of Miami

The most comprehensive program of massage-related research is the University of Miami's Touch Research Institute. Created in 1991 by the school of medicine, it is the world's first center for basic and applied research in the use of touch in human health and development. Directed by Tiffany Field, Ph.D., a professor of psychology, pediatrics, and psychiatry, the TRI has a multidisciplinary staff of forty scientists from the fields of medicine, biology, and psychology and another thirty visiting scientists from other universities participating in collaborative studies.

A plethora of studies have demonstrated impressive benefits

for integrating massage therapy into medical care. In one study, premature infants treated with daily massage therapy gained 47 percent more weight per day and had shorter hospital stays by six days than those that were not massaged, resulting in cost savings of approximately $3000 per infant.[12]

Jason

Jason, fifty-five, was suffering from pain in both hips, which had become arthritic. He had been very athletic most of his life, running and playing basketball and tennis. He had been told by a physician that he may be facing a hip replacement as his condition had been degenerating over several years—particularly in the right hip.

He sought the help of Bridget Beck, a Rolfer in Santa Rosa, California, who gave him the standard series of ten Rolfing sessions. Beck observed that he had an external rotation of the right leg (turning outward), a rotation of the pelvis, and an unequal distribution of weight on his legs. The rotator muscles in his buttocks were chronically tight in order to support this pattern and all of this resulted in more stress to the hip joints.

The Rolfing balanced the pelvis and brought the right leg back into alignment with the hip joint to allow more proper tracking through the motion of the joint. His weight became properly distributed over both legs.

He also gained more flexibility and balance to all the segments of his body. He reported greater ease of movement, more vitality, and reduction in hip joint pain to where he was able to return to sports activity. At one point he asked if he might be misusing the Rolfing by becoming so active again.

A study of the effects of massage therapy on HIV patients found that those who received a massage five times a week for one month had higher numbers of natural killer (NK) cells, which were also more potent. They also had less anxiety and lower serotonin (stress hormone) levels.[13]

A third study involved giving massage therapy to fifty-two hospitalized depressed and adjustment disordered children and adolescents. A separate comparison group viewed relaxation videotapes. Those receiving the massage therapy were less depressed and anxious and had lower saliva cortisol levels, which is an indicator of less depression. [14]

Following is a list of other applications of massage therapy currently being studied at TRI:

- Newborns of cocaine-addicted mothers
- HIV-exposed newborns
- Infants of depressed mothers
- Infant colic
- Infant sleep disorders
- Infants with cancer
- Preschool children
- Neglected children
- Abused children
- Autistic children
- Posttraumatic stress disorder after Hurricane Andrew
- Pediatric skin disorders
- Asthma
- Diabetes
- Juvenile rheumatoid arthritis
- Depressed teenage mothers
- Teenage mothers' childbirth labor
- Eating disorders
- Job performance/stress
- Pregnancy
- Hypertension
- HIV and improved immune function
- Spinal cord injuries
- Fibromyalgia syndrome

- Rape and spouse abuse
- Couples' sex therapy
- Volunteer foster grandparents
- Arthritis
- Chronic fatigue syndrome

Bodywork Research

Little research has been conducted on the various forms of bodywork. One exception is Rolfing, for which several studies have found interesting effects.

In one controlled study, forty-eight participants were randomly assigned to either the experimental group (Rolfing) or a control group (no Rolfing). A significant decrease in anxiety was found in those who received the treatment over a five-week period. The researchers explained these findings in terms of the theory that the Rolfing caused a release of emotional tension that had been stored up in the muscles, which in turn resulted in lower anxiety scores on a psychological test of state anxiety.[15]

Other studies of Rolfing have found improvements in muscular efficiency,[16] reductions in anxiety,[17] decrease in pelvic tilt, and increase in vagal tone (amplitude of respiratory sinus arrhythmia, a heart rate function that corresponds with reduced stress in the body).[18]

STRENGTHS AND LIMITATIONS

Massage therapy and bodywork obviously have a very broad, diverse range of applications. Essentially, they can support any health condition that would benefit from greater blood circulation and the release of tension. Psychological conditions also are affected beneficially, as the physiological changes that occur with these kinds of intervention help harmonize and rebalance the nervous and hormonal systems.

There is great potential in using massage to reduce cumulative traumatic disorders in the workplace. For example, chicken cutters in chicken processing plants often develop carpal tunnel problems. Several companies in the chicken processing industry in Virginia have developed worksite massage programs that have shown impressive reductions in these problems. The most frequently used techniques include cross-fiber, deep tissue, and Swedish, concentrated on those muscle groups that are chronically stressed in the work (hands, arms, shoulders, and back). The programs also teach self-massage techniques and the results include better morale and reduced absenteeism.

Contraindications to massage or bodywork are few and may include transmittable skin diseases, unhealed wounds, postoperative conditions, and blood clots. In many cases, of course, such therapy can avoid problem areas in the body, assuming the practitioner is aware of the condition.

Many people wonder about whether massage or bodywork could cause a cancer to metastasize. According to Elliot Greene, "This is an area where research is needed to define the risk. Practitioners are generally taught to err on the side of conservatism. For example, massage is not recommended for someone immediately after chemotherapy or radiation treatment.

"Physiologically, it is not easy to metastasize a tumor from simple pressure and studies have shown that the body has a number of layers of defenses to prevent that from happening simply from touch. It is known, however, that certain kinds of chemotherapies in particular make the tissue fragile for a couple of days and massage immediately after such therapies might irritate the tissues. If there was any danger of metastasizing, it would be more likely to happen closer to the treatment. A conservative response would be to use much lighter forms of massage."[19]

In fact, massage therapy is increasingly being incorporated into complementary cancer therapy programs. At the Cancer Support and Education Center in Menlo Park, California, it has been an integral part of a program that resulted in significant improvement in quality of life, even for patients with metastatic disease.[20]

The ability of massage to reduce anxiety, depression, and stress is a logical counter to the strain a cancer patient must deal with in facing a life-threatening condition and traumatic treatment.

THE PRACTITIONER-PATIENT RELATIONSHIP

Hands-on therapies naturally foster a kind of intimacy between the practitioner and patient. In many of the approaches, the recipient partially or fully disrobes and lies on a table (though they are draped with a sheet and are never fully exposed), which further contributes to the intimacy and vulnerability that may be felt when using this tradition. Normal boundaries of social interaction are crossed. Hence there is a special need for sensitivity and regard for the client on the part of the practitioner that matches and perhaps even exceeds that of many doctor-patient relationships.

There is a wide range of attitudes among practitioners about how they view their role. Some think of themselves as healers or therapists, working with the whole person through the body. Certain approaches (e.g., the Rosen Method) are explicitly focused on engaging the person on the emotional level and working with emotional issues in the context of the body with subtle verbal suggestions. Others may take a more mechanistic approach toward working with the body. They may not wish to engage the client on the emotional level at all but rather concentrate on physical techniques. Some see themselves as facilitators, some as educators.

There is wide variation among practitioners, even *within* the specific approaches, as to how much verbal exchange takes place and the degree to which the practitioner is available for emotional or psychological support.

Finally, some approaches require a series of sessions over a

A Doctor's Story

A patient was brought to our intensive care unit from another hospital emergency room, where he had been given a hundred milligrams of Thorazine (an antipsychotic drug) intramuscularly. Thorazine has a faster and greater effect when injected than when taken orally, but it also has a greater chance of lowering the blood pressure. This man had been given a very high dosage—and they hadn't noticed that he was drunk. You *never* mix alcohol and major antipsychotics because they are additive in effect.

When the patient arrived, the medication was just taking effect. He went under before the eyes of the admitting personnel, becoming less responsive and groggy, then turning gray. When I arrived, the pulse was so weak that I couldn't feel it and the blood pressure was 40/0, which indicates a coronary arrest with the imminent danger of croaking. By the time we got him into a room, he was totally unresponsive and just whitish gray, like a person looks just before dying due to lack of oxygen.

I put my knuckle into his sternum and dug in hard to elicit a pain reflex and stimulate adrenaline release, which sometimes can revive a person. Nothing. I didn't have the necessary medical equipment to do some of the things that Western medicine can do because this was a psychiatric unit. Here I was, looking at a guy who was going to have a cardiac arrest at any moment. I could stand by and watch him die or I could do something—anything. I suddenly remembered . . . a primary revival point and the most important one for loss of consciousness. So I pulled the patient's shoes off and, without explaining to the nurses what I was doing, proceeded to put my thumbs almost through his feet at these points.

It took about two minutes, three at the most. He

started moving around a bit at first and then moaning
a little. By the end of those few minutes, he had sat up
in his chair and was talking to us. He had a strong
pulse and a blood pressure of 90/40. There was an
amazed look on the nurses' faces as they asked what I
had done. I said I had worked with the acupressure
points to mobilize reserve energy. I don't know if that
made any sense to them, but they were amazed and
happy that the patient was alive. Meanwhile, by the
way, a priority code ambulance—with sirens and lights
and the whole bit—was on its way to pick up a suppos-
edly dying patient.[21]

period of time (e.g., Rolfing, Hellerwork), which naturally fosters a therapeutic relationship and requires communication, instruction, and feedback. On the other hand, many European or
Western forms of massage are complete in themselves as one
session and do not really require any communication between
practitioner and client. It is not unusual to experience an entire
massage without a word being spoken.

EVALUATING PERSONAL RESULTS

The subjective experience of the client is generally the most
important way of evaluating personal results. However, sometimes the change process naturally causes temporary discomfort,
which needs to be accepted, so that expectations of feeling good
may not always be appropriate.

Practitioners of the various methods can often also give the
client feedback based on what they feel through their hands and
what they see with their eyes.

Some modalities, particularly those of structural/functional/ movement integration, use visual feedback in the form of having clients look at themselves in mirrors or even taking "before and after" photographs. The photographic record is particularly common in Rolfing and Hellerwork as a way of following progress over time.

Some of the movement integration therapies also use videotape to help observe changes in function, posture, and range of motion.

RELATIONSHIP TO OTHER FORMS OF MEDICINE

These modalities tend to be highly complementary to all other medical traditions. They can enhance the effectiveness of other forms of treatment by inducing relaxation, promoting circulation, and their other common benefits. They can also help patients tolerate more invasive approaches and handle the side effects of other treatments.

COSTS

Costs tend to be higher in urban areas. Generally, the cost of massage therapy will range from $30 to $60 for an hour and will be somewhat lower in less urban environments. Cost of other more specialized modalities may be higher. Rolfing, for example, averages around $75 to $80 for a ninety-minute session and is ordinarily done in a series of ten sessions spaced at least a week apart.

Other modalities tend to fall within these ranges. Most insurance companies do not cover massage and bodywork, although such coverage is much more likely if it is prescribed by a physician. Massage therapy is more likely to be covered than the other methods, although a physician's prescription and the licensure of the practitioner may help increase the chances.

CHOOSING A PRACTITIONER

Massage Therapy

Massage therapists are designated by a variety of titles, some referring to state regulation and others to other forms of certification. Various counties and cities may also have ordinances regulating the practice of massage.

It should be noted that practitioners of many health care disciplines often learn some massage therapy techniques during the course of their training without necessarily having any of the following credentials. Thus they may practice massage therapy (and facilitate insurance coverage) under another kind of license or credential such as nursing, chiropractic, or the like.

The AMTA has recently begun to discourage practitioners from using initials after their names, feeling this may be confusing to the public because there is no standardization and such initials tend to mimic academic degrees. Instead the AMTA encourages practitioners to spell out what their credential is. In some states the use of initials is controlled (such as licensed massage therapist, L.M.T.), but in many states it is meaningless.

The most common titles for massage therapists are as follows:

Nationally Certified in Therapeutic Massage and Bodywork. This title designates the person has completed the requirements for and passed the National Certification Board for Therapeutic Massage and Bodywork (N.C.B.T.M.B.). This is the leading national certification exam.

Massage Practitioner (M.P.). This title is often used by practitioners whose training is less extensive than that required for certification by schools or by the AMTA as a massage therapist.

Certified Massage Therapist (C.M.T.). This is a voluntary, professional, nongovernmental certification from organizations that can attest to the therapist's competency. This is granted by many massage therapy schools, which may or may not meet AMTA standards for training. Thus the quality of this credential depends on the quality of the certifier and its standards. (For example, even a person who has only taken an eight-hour course can claim to be certified.)

Registered Massage Therapist (R.M.T.). This is a form of voluntary licensing for the use of a specific professional title. Rarely used in the United States, some Canadian provinces use this to designate government licensing. At one time it also designated a special credential for members of the AMTA who had advanced training in therapeutic massage and passed a special exam, but this usage has been discontinued.

Licensed Massage Therapist (L.M.T.). This refers to occupational licensing by a state or local government. Nineteen states have licensing laws requiring massage therapists to meet minimum standards of training. The basic requirement is usually five hundred hours of classroom training with instructors present, followed by a written and practical exam. The following states have licensing laws: Arkansas, Connecticut, Delaware, Florida, Hawaii, Iowa, Louisiana, Maine, Nebraska, New Hampshire, New Mexico, New York, North Dakota, Ohio, Oregon, Rhode Island, Tennessee, Texas, Utah, and Washington, D.C.

In states that do not require licensing, a good credential to seek is graduation from an AMTA-accredited program that meets the five hundred–hour standard. There are many schools of massage therapy and bodywork that require fewer hours of training (often one hundred to two hundred hours), so the extent of training is an important question in choosing a practitioner.

The American Massage Therapy Association is the predominant organization for massage therapists with over eighteen thousand members, representing all fifty states, D.C., the Virgin Islands, and several foreign countries. Membership is a good

A Case of "Broken-Hearted Feet"

Amy was a fifty-year-old woman who came to a Rosen Method practitioner for help with a variety of stress-related symptoms in her body. She was particularly concerned about a sensation that the bones in her feet were crumbling, though there was no physical indication of this. She had several sessions over a period of months.

During the course of one session the practitioner asked her what happened to the free, fun-loving little girl that she once was. This stimulated Amy's recall of an experience of riding her horse all around and being free. She then remembered that one day during her adolescence her parents, without warning, sold her beloved horse. She recalled that the horse had bad feet. The practitioner commented, "It's interesting about the horse's feet . . ." At this, Amy began to experience a welling up of deep feelings of unexpressed grief at the loss of her horse, feelings she hadn't been able to express before.

Gail Gardener, a Rosen Method practitioner in Sebastopol, California, recounts this story as an example of how bodywork can help bring to awareness previously unexpressed feelings, resulting in their release.

indication of professional preparation. It requires one of the following:

1. Graduation from a training program approved by the Commission on Massage Training Accreditation/Approval. This is an accreditation agency commissioned by the AMTA. This assures the practitioner has completed a

program of a minimum of six months duration with five hundred in-class hours of training. There are currently fifty-eight massage therapy schools accredited by COMTAA. Subjects include anatomy and physiology, massage techniques, and practical training.

2. Holding a state license that meets AMTA certification standards.
3. Passing an AMTA membership entrance examination.
4. Passing the National Certification Examination for Therapeutic Massage and Bodywork. Six states have adopted this exam, developed by the AMTA, as their licensing exam. It is anticipated that eventually all the states that license massage will adopt this exam and the number of such states is expected to increase.

   In early 1994 this exam was accredited by the National Commission for Certifying Agencies, a major independent agency that evaluates professional certification programs according to stringent standards.

Membership in the AMTA also requires six hours of continuing education every two years.

The AMTA publishes a membership registry for use by its members and provides referrals to local practitioners. Address: 820 Davis St., Suite 100, Evanston, IL 60201–4444, phone (708) 864–0123.

Other Forms of Bodywork or Energy Work

Finding a competent practitioner of the other forms of bodywork or energy work is essentially a matter of asking whether they are certified by the particular professional association for the method being used. Some practitioners integrate multiple methods, but if they are not certified in any one, their preparation is dubious. It is best to work with someone who has completed training and thereby has achieved a standard of expertise in at least one method.

Following are the professional associations for the most common forms of bodywork and energy work.

Rolf Institute of Structural Integration. The training is typically twelve months long for basic certification. A Certified Advanced Rolfer is one who has practiced at least five years and has taken an additional six weeks training. A list of certified practitioners is available. Address: 205 Canyon Blvd., Boulder, CO 80302, phone (800) 530–8875.

Hellerwork, Inc. Training is a 1,250-hour program leading to certification as a Hellerwork practitioner. Trainings are offered internationally. Address: 406 Berry St., Mt. Shasta, CA 96067, phone (800) 392–3900 or (916) 926–2500.

Rosen Method Professional Association. Certification training is two years plus an eighteen-month internship. Certified practitioners must also hold a state-approved massage certificate. A directory of practitioners is available from the association. Address: 2550 Shattuck Ave., Box 49, Berkeley, CA 94704, phone (510) 644–4166.

The Trager Institute. Training for Trager practitioners takes a minimum of 269 hours usually over at least six months. A list of certified practitioners is available. Address: 33 Millwood St., Mill Valley, CA 94941, phone (415) 388–2688, FAX (415) 388–2710.

The Feldenkrais Guild. Only people trained by Moshe Feldenkrais or graduates of guild accredited training programs are eligible to be members of the guild. Practitioner members are qualified teachers of Awareness Through Movement and Functional Integration. Associate members are qualified teachers of Awareness Through Movement. The professional training program spans 160 days over three and a half years. The guild publishes a directory of certified practitioners. Address: 706 Ellsworth St., P.O. Box 489, Albany, OR 97321–0143, phone (800) 775–2118 or (503) 926–0981.

North American Society of Teachers of the Alexander Technique (NASTAT) formed in 1987 to educate the public about the Alexander Technique, to establish and maintain standards

Marianne

Marianne had injured her neck several months ago but still had so much pain that she could not tolerate having it touched or moved. She was seeing a physical therapist but her sensitivity to pain prevented her from receiving much of the routine physical therapy care that was indicated for her injury.

She received a Jin Shin Jyutsu session that lasted one hour with extremely light contact on her neck. After the session her pain increased slightly, but the next morning it was less than half of what it had been and she could begin to move her neck.

According to Joanna Chieppa, a practitioner in Sonoma County, CA, with this type of work often there is an immediate decrease in pain. Occasionally, however, the client may experience a temporary increase in pain as more energy moves through an area that is inflamed or blocked. Once the blockage is cleared this brief discomfort is typically followed by a significant improvement in symptoms.

After Marianne's next session two days later there was no increase in pain and she felt even greater relief. Within two weeks she could move her neck freely, had minimal pain, and was able to receive and benefit from the prescribed physical therapy.

for certification of teachers and teacher training courses in the United States, and to ensure that the educational principles of the Alexander Technique are upheld. It publishes a directory of certified teachers. Training to become a teacher takes three years (sixteen hundred hours). Address: P.O. Box 112484, Tacoma, WA 98411–2484, phone (800) 473–0620 or (206) 627–3766.

Nurse Healers Professional Associates, Inc., provides information about Therapeutic Touch and training for health care providers. The length of trainings varies and there is no formal certification. Address: P.O. Box 444, Allison Park, PA 15101, phone (412) 355–8476.

Jin Shin Jyutsu, Inc., is an organization for practitioners who have completed a five-day training course in this method. Practitioners are encouraged to repeat the basic training several times, but there is no formal certification. There is also an advanced course. Address: 8719 E. San Alberto, Scottsdale, AZ 85258, phone (602) 998–9331.

Jin Shin Do® Foundation for Bodymind Acupressure™ is a network of authorized teachers and registered practitioners who have received standardized training in this approach. Registered practitioners have 250 hours of training plus practical experience. A directory of registered practitioners and authorized teachers is available from the foundation. Address: 366 California Ave., Suite 16, Palo Alto, CA 94306, or P.O. Box 1097, Felton, CA 95018, or call J.S.D.F. in Palo Alto, CA at (415) 328–1811.

American Oriental Bodywork Therapy Association (AOBTA) is an educational and certifying organization for practitioners of a variety of forms of oriental bodywork. Associate members have at least 150 hours of training with a certified instructor and a hundred hours of practice. Certified practitioners have completed five hundred hours of such training and passed a certification exam. AOBTA has about eight hundred members and publishes a membership directory. Address: 6801 Jericho Turnpike, Syosset, NY 11791, phone (516) 364–5533.

Associated Bodywork and Massage Professionals (ABMP) provides professional support and legislative advocacy for massage therapists and bodyworkers. Membership is of two levels: practitioner level requires a hundred hours of training. Professional level requires five hundred hours or state licensure or registration. ABMP also publishes *Massage and Bodywork Quarterly*. Address: 28677 Buffalo Park Rd., Evergreen CO 80439, phone (303) 674–8478.

The Upledger Institute, Inc., is an educational and clinical resource and training center for manipulative therapies such as CranioSacral Therapy™, visceral manipulation, and other holistically oriented approaches used by bodyworkers. Founded by John Upledger, D.O., it conducts training nationally and internationally. It also produces several instructional publications and a directory of alumni of its trainings. Address: 11211 Prosperity Farms Rd., Palm Beach Gardens, FL 33410, phone (800) 233–5880.

American Academy of Reflexology conducts training in ear, hand, and foot reflexology and can provide referrals to certified practitioners. Address: 606 E. Magnolia Blvd., Suite B, Burbank, CA 91501, phone (818) 841–7741.

International Institute of Reflexology conducts two-day trainings nationally and internationally and a certification exam in the Ingham Method of reflexology. They also can provide referrals to trained practitioners. Address: 5650 First Avenue North, P.O. Box 12642, St. Petersburg, FL 33733, phone (813) 343–4811.

Zero Balancing Association offers training in this method, a fifty-hour basic course, and an eighteen-month certification program. Address: P.O. Box 1727, Capitola, CA 95010, phone (408) 476–0665.

CHAPTER 10

NEW CHOICES, NEW REALITIES

"The turn of the last century proved to be a watershed in science; it coincided with the beginnings of the new physics. This one happens to be the turn of a whole millennium. I hope philosophers of the twenty-second century will be able to look back on it as the beginning of the new medicine."

—ANDREW WEIL, M.D.[1]

Our purpose to this point has been to survey the differences among the various traditions in the service of making an informed choice. You may feel a general sense of resonance with a particular tradition. Or you may base your choices on other criteria such as the special expertise of a certain practitioner, the importance of being touched, economic considerations, or a feeling of greater confidence in the more scientifically documented approaches.

There are three broad dimensions of treatment by which we can compare and contrast the different traditions. These involve their orientations toward *somatic, herbal and nutritional,* and *energetic* approaches. The *somatic* approaches are those which have the practitioner or patient working directly with the physical body through some form of physical contact or movement. The *herbal and nutritional* approaches are less direct and work

307

by nourishing the tissues of the body with herbs or nutrients. The *energetic* therapies are more subtle still, working with the energy field or energy systems of the person. The table on pages 310–11 presents a comparison of the role of each of these dimensions within each tradition.

There is much overlap among the three dimensions, as many of the therapies fit into more than one category. For example, both manipulation and herbs are sometimes used to influence energy.

There are myriad other criteria that can also be considered for choosing among traditions. In stepping back to look at the big picture, however, there are two additional dimensions that bear further reflection. One is the question of *who* provides the actual treatment, practitioner or patient. The other is the matter of our culturally conditioned expectations about the *time* involved in any healing process.

Who's in Charge?

The variety of medical traditions can be thought of as positioned along a continuum, with one end representing complete reliance on the expertise of a practitioner for healing and the other end representing complete reliance on the behavior of the patient. In the middle would be traditions requiring some sort of interdependence between the efforts of the practitioner and those of the patient.

For many people, one of the greatest motives in choosing alternative medicine is the desire to take a greater degree of control over their health, to have a greater sense of self-determination and involvement. Not everyone is equally interested in this motive, however. Some prefer alternative therapies on the basis of their being nontoxic or noninvasive, but still prefer to be treated rather than to be part of the treatment themselves through changing how they live.

For example, the success of classical homeopathy, like that of allopathy, is dependent on the practitioner's skill in determining the right remedy. Little is required of the patient other than perhaps avoiding certain antidoting substances. Likewise, while a chiropractor or osteopath may suggest certain exercises or other lifestyle changes, skillfully applied manipulations by the practitioner may still be considered the key to alleviating a particular problem. Acupuncture, massage therapy, and bodywork are also primarily dependent on the practitioner for their results.

On the other hand Chinese herbs, Ayurveda, many naturopathic approaches, and mind/body medicine depend a great deal more on the patient's full participation. The practitioner may serve more as a consultant or teacher (the original meaning of "doctor") than as a treater or healer and give guidelines for daily self-treatment.

The success of these approaches is much more dependent on the active involvement of the patient. Whether it is mixing herbs at specified times each day, complying with dietary guidelines, using hydrotherapy on a regular schedule, or daily practice of the relaxation response, health benefits from these approaches depend on the cumulative effects of the person's behavior. It takes time to do these things. It may require a reordering of priorities and may at times be inconvenient.

This raises the question of how willing we actually are to participate fully in our own health. The payoffs of course can include a sense of accomplishment, self-esteem, self-empowerment, and pride when good results are achieved.

A Matter of Time

The alternative medical traditions can be thought of as sharing a vitalistic orientation—that is, they all presuppose that there is a life force or vital energy involved in healing. One issue that commonly arises in choosing any such tradition is the question of how long it takes and our cultural preoccupation with time urgency.

309

Therapeutic Approaches of Alternative Medical Traditions

TRADITION	SOMATIC APPROACHES	HERBAL AND NUTRITIONAL APPROACHES	ENERGETIC APPROACHES
CHINESE MEDICINE	Acupressure Other oriental massage *Chi kung* Tai chi	Chinese herbs Dietary guidance	Acupuncture Moxabustion Acupressure Tai chi *Chi kung*
AYURVEDA	Massage *Pranayama* Yoga	Ayurvedic herbs Dietary guidance	*Pranayama* Massage Meditation
HOMEOPATHY	None	None	Homeopathic remedies
NATUROPATHIC MEDICINE	Variety of manipulative therapies, massage and bodywork Hydrotherapy	Both Eastern and Western herbal medicine Dietary guidance	May use methods from all traditions
MIND/BODY MEDICINE	Exercise, yoga, *chi kung*, tai chi, and other self-directed practices	Compliance with dietary guidelines provided by other traditions	Imagery Biofeedback Relaxation

			Meditation Breath therapy Chi kung, tai chi Autogenic training Hypnosis Psychotherapy Group support
OSTEOPATHIC MEDICINE	Osteopathic manipulation of all the bones, tissues and organs of the body	Depends on the individual practitioner's training and interests	Depends on the individual practitioner's training and interests
CHIROPRACTIC	Chiropractic manipulation of skeletal system and soft tissue	Depends on the individual practitioner's training and interests	Depends on the individual practitioner's training and interests
MASSAGE THERAPY and BODYWORK	Traditional European Contemporary Western Structural Functional Movement integration Oriental Energetic (nonoriental) Other approaches	None	Energetic methods of bodywork (oriental and nonoriental)

We westerners are living in an era of fast food, fast cars, and fast medicine. By growing up with allopathy, we have learned to expect instantaneous results. Pharmaceutical drugs and surgery, which lie outside the vitalistic paradigm of healing, are designed to achieve rapid elimination of the body's symptoms. The vitalistically oriented traditions operate on a different principle, one that usually requires the passage of time as the body's self-repair mechanisms reestablish homeostasis.

While chiropractic, osteopathy, and bodywork sometimes achieve impressive results instantaneously, often a longer process over time is required. Likewise, homeopathy can sometimes bring spectacular results immediately. More commonly, however, it too is more involved, requiring perhaps several tries to find the right remedy and maybe also the taking of a daily dose.

Naturopathy, Chinese medicine, Ayurveda, and mind/body medicine tend also to require patience in order for tangible results to take hold. These approaches rely on using the body's inherent healing responses to build momentum to restore health. They excel with chronic illnesses that have taken a long time to evolve, but they do take time. Some practitioners even have formulas for estimating how long it takes to recover from a given condition based on how long it took the condition to develop.

From the vitalistic perspective, healing is a process that builds momentum over time—somewhat like boiling a pot of water. When we want to boil water, we place the pot over a source of heat, check to see that the heat source is properly supplied with fuel, and wait patiently for the water to reach the boiling point. We have no trouble accepting the fact that we cannot rush the process and that it simply takes time for the water to reach the boiling point. We do not throw out the stove and buy another one because it is not performing as quickly as we would like.

In the same way, working within a vitalistic paradigm requires a different orientation toward time than we have when using allopathy. In some cases, particularly in chronic illnesses, a given treatment process may take weeks or even months to achieve the results we want. Thus patience is required a great deal more with most alternative traditions than with allopathy.

312

On Choosing

Imagine you have a certain symptom that could easily be eliminated in one week by taking a pharmaceutical drug three times a day. The drug has some side effects, but they are tolerable. Its long-term effects on your vital energy and immune system are unknown. Still, the convenience is attractive, it has been proven effective in controlled studies, and it is approved by the FDA.

Now imagine you are offered a naturopathic approach that only takes three days. It is drug-free and has also been found effective in controlled studies. Sounds great, but it requires you to interrupt your schedule to carry out a time-consuming routine of boiling up an herbal concoction twice each day plus taking a daily hydrotherapy treatment in your bathtub.

Which would you choose? Perhaps you opt for the naturopathic approach, thinking that you really believe in natural healing whenever possible and you'd like to reduce the amount of drugs in your life. Now suppose you are informed this same regime must be carried out daily for two weeks in order to get the same result as the drug. Or how about four weeks? Where would you draw the line?

BUILDING BRIDGES: INTEGRATIVE MEDICINE

Just as every religion has had fundamentalists who believe their worldview is the only valid one and all who differ are living in darkness, every medical tradition has also had them. None has been immune to the propensity to label other traditions as irresponsible, harmful, or quackery. Fortunately, such fundamen-

313

talism is on the decline as it has become clear that no single tradition has all the answers for the emerging health challenges we face.

We now know that at least a third of Americans use some form of alternative medicine. On their own, people are choosing to integrate other traditions with their regular allopathic care. By voting with their feet, they are choosing a new paradigm of health care that could be called *integrative medicine.*

The lay public is far ahead of the health care establishment in embracing this new paradigm. Some people routinely use a combination of alternative approaches. Others integrate other traditions with allopathic medicine and, according to the Eisenberg study, do not bother to reveal this to their M.D.s.

As we have seen throughout this book, many practitioners of alternative medicine are themselves trained in multiple traditions and create their own version of integrative medicine. However, a growing number of mainstream practitioners are also incorporating other approaches. It is likely that the greatest number of practitioners of alternative medicine in the United States will eventually be allopathically trained physicians.

Many already use nutritional and herbal therapies drawn from naturopathic or oriental principles. Homeopathy, mind/body approaches, and, to a lesser degree, manipulative therapies and acupuncture are drawing new adherents.

A growing number use conventional procedures (lab tests or high-tech tests) to arrive at a diagnosis but then use nonallopathic approaches for treatment. In cases of acute illness, advanced disease, or emergency situations they may incorporate pharmaceutical drugs or surgery—the real strengths of allopathy—with these other approaches.

In short, they use allopathy and alternative approaches in a complementary relationship. They take an attitude that transcends the divisions among traditions and describe their philosophy as "whatever works."

This often allows them to take the uniqueness of the patient more into account. Since different traditions have different ways of defining and thinking about symptoms, a patient may not "fit any categories" of one tradition, while they may fit perfectly

HIV: Cracking the Nut

"I see HIV as the condition that 'cracks the nut' of standard Western care being 'unidimensional,' " says Jon Kaiser, M.D. "This is such a fascinating, complex, challenging condition that the only thing that's going to work is integrative medicine. The virus is so adept at adjusting to whatever drugs are thrown at it that what has been the most successful in keeping it at bay is the body's own strong immune response.

"I believe very strongly in the body's healing mechanisms. When I started the work, I hoped that by just using natural therapies I would be successful in the majority of cases. I *believed* that any individual, given the right mix of nutrients, exercise, and stress reduction could tap in to strengthening their immune system.

"What I learned was that a percentage of individuals could do that, using that limited model. However, I found that there was an enormous amount of emotional disease in many of these patients. I wondered whether focusing on healing or clearing up some of this would have a positive effect on immune function. In fact, based on my experience, it is of paramount importance that one address that issue.

"Then I figured acting in *both* of these areas would be enough to tap into the healing mechanisms and keep people stable. My experience has been that in a large number of patients that is true, but there are still a number of people, either due to deep-rooted conflicts, an extremely virulent viral condition, or a genetically weaker immune system, for whom medications are necessary *as an adjunct to everything else.*"[15]

into a category of another tradition, giving a perfectly clear set of treatment guidelines.

For example, what might appear to be a set of vague, non-disease-specific symptoms to a conventional allopath may be clearly a case of *vata* imbalance to an integrative physician who can draw upon Ayurvedic principles. Clear guidelines for diet and behavior change would follow. While chronic fatigue syndrome continues to perplex allopathy, in Chinese medicine it is clearly a *chi* deficiency disorder.

An illustration of the advantages of true versatility is offered by Elson Haas, M.D., of the Preventive Medical Centers of Marin and Sonoma in San Rafael and Cotati, California. Haas's clinics include an osteopath, nurse practitioner, massage therapists and bodyworkers, acupuncturists, homeopaths, physical therapist, nutritional counselor, and a hypnotherapist.

Haas himself uses naturopathic, Chinese, and allopathic approaches. He describes treating a woman with acute bronchitis/laryngitis: "She was going on a trip in a couple days. Because this was an acute situation and she doesn't get sick very often, I wrote a prescription for amoxicillin (an antibiotic), the simplest, quickest thing to do. If we were to work in a more natural approach—start dealing with why she's sick and how she takes care of herself—I couldn't get her better as quickly.

"Allopathy's great when the situation is 'I'm ailing right now, just get me back in the ball game as quickly as possible.' But if people get recurrently ill and you just keep treating symptoms, you actually make them sicker over the long run. It works well in crisis management, but it's really very weak in chronic problems."

Earlier chapters discussed several important studies of integrated approaches to what are symbolically our most pressing crises—heart disease, cancer, and AIDS. To review:

The program for reversing heart disease developed by Dean Ornish, M.D., at the Preventive Medicine Research Institute at the University of California, San Francisco, uses diet and moderate exercise (consistent with naturopathic principles); stress management, meditation, and participation in a weekly support group (mind/body medicine); yoga; and monitoring by allo-

Allopathy's New Nemesis: Drug Resistance

In May 1993 a group of prominent researchers at the annual meeting of the American Society of Microbiology in Atlanta declared that the world is facing a medical crisis from diseases that have become resistant to the antibiotics most commonly used to treat them. Such diseases as tuberculosis, gonorrhea, meningitis, pneumonia, and food poisoning are no longer effectively treated with drugs that had been used successfully for decades.

The experts attribute this growing problem to worldwide patterns of misuse or overuse of so-called miracle drug antibiotics—such as giving them to children for preventive purposes (as in day care); using them in common illnesses such as flu, when they are unnecessary and can damage the body's naturally occurring healthful bacteria; and using broad-spectrum antibiotics that also kill healthful organisms in the body.

The common staphylococcus bacteria is now resistant to all antibiotics except vancomycin. According to Dr. Alexander Tomasz of Rockefeller University, "It's only a matter of time until staphylococcus becomes resistant to vancomycin, and then we will have no way to treat these infections." He adds, "We are playing a dangerous chess game with these organisms and it is a game we are very close to losing."[16]

pathic diagnostic procedures, with conventional drugs only on an as-needed basis.

At UCLA and Stanford medical schools, studies found improved survival in malignant melanoma and metastatic breast cancer patients who used group mind/body medicine programs along with regular medical care. In China, several studies of

Chinese herbs used in combination with chemotherapy or radiation also reported improvements in survival rates for several types of cancer.

In working with HIV, San Francisco physician Jon Kaiser, M.D., uses a combination of naturopathic approaches, mind/body medicine, and allopathic drugs to achieve a remarkable 89-percent rate of either keeping HIV patients stable or actually improving their diagnosis. Such work not only helps maintain a good quality of life for the individual but also buys critical time in which a vaccine or other treatments could be developed.

Indeed, Jonas Salk, M.D., and others have found what they consider to be promising indications that such a vaccine may not be far off. If and when such a vaccine is developed, however, there will still be a need for integrative approaches since a vaccine will not be a panacea for all those affected by this disease.

According to Kaiser, "The biggest mistake of standard Western medicine is to go to nutrition, stress reduction, and psychotherapy *when the drugs don't work*, after you get to the end of the line. It's a more effective model by far to *start* with a strong program of natural therapies and emotional healing and *then* reach for the drugs, as a last resort or as necessary after that."[2]

Among the most popular champions of integrative medicine is Andrew Weil, M.D., Director of the Program in Integrative Medicine at the University of Arizona Medical School. In his very successful book *Spontaneous Healing* (Knopf, 1995), he proposes a new kind of health care institution—one that would be more like a spa than a hospital, integrating the best ideas of both conventional and alternative medicine. Patients would learn and practice the principles of healthy living and would be partners with their health professionals rather than dependent upon them.

Further he proposes that medical education be overhauled—that medical students be taught alternative models of science and health, study the healing power of nature, and be encouraged to develop themselves into healthy role models for their patients. Weil is a visionary whose ideas point clearly to a new direction for medicine.

CONCLUSION

Among the ancient Tibetan prophecies is recorded a vision of a time in which human beings would forget how to live a life of health and harmony. They would become absorbed in the production and consumption of material things and would be preoccupied with outward productivity and materialism. Their minds would be busy, confused, and agitated.

Their culture would produce many "evil artificial substances" that poison the air, earth, water, food, and the people themselves. They would suffer from a category of illnesses the Tibetans called *nyen* diseases, which would be attributable to lifestyle, technology, and environmental pollution.[3]

Indeed, we are now seeing both the emergence of new diseases and a stubborn resurgence of old ones. The compelling need for a widespread integration of the strengths of all traditions is obvious when we consider the new disease patterns and our changing environment.

A recent article in the *Journal of the American Medical Association* concluded that nearly half of all deaths occurring in America are premature.[4] Granted, allopathy has made significant inroads against some chronic and degenerative diseases, but the fact remains that overall the trends are still growing.

More than one in four of us have some form of heart or circulatory disease, which remains the leading cause of death. However, if recent trends continue, cancer will surpass heart disease as the leading cause of death in just a few years.[5] Other conditions that are becoming increasingly prevalent include chronic lung diseases,[6] tuberculosis,[7] hepatitis B,[8] Alzheimer's disease,[9] diabetes mellitus and end-stage renal disease,[10] bowel diseases,[11] chronic migraine headaches,[12] Lyme disease,[13] chronic fatigue syndrome, fibromyalgia, and environmental illnesses.

As for the changing environment, recent years have seen enormous changes that are bound to affect us individually and on a mass scale.

- Urbanization and crowding bring us into contact with an ever-diversifying pool of viruses, bacteria, and other pathogens.
- The economic problems of access to primary care and preventive services result in a growing pool of people with compromised host resistance and greater exposure to opportunistic diseases.
- Immigration and international commerce are constantly adding to the diversity of pathogens we must encounter.
- Industry introduces billions of pounds of toxic pollutants into the atmosphere annually.[14]
- The expansion of populated areas into animal habitats promotes cross-species transfer of pathogens, both to humans and their pets.
- International tourism and the mass transit of military personnel into new environments (such as the Persian Gulf and Somalia), followed by their abrupt return, helps introduce new pathogens into the general population.

Clearly our health as individuals does not exist in isolation. The inner ecology of the body depends on the ability of the greater environment to sustain it. As stated by Leonard Duhl, M.D., professor of public health at the University of California, Berkeley, "No matter how good our medicine is, it will still not keep us healthy if we are immersed in a toxic environment."

We also dare not overlook the fact that the social crises of poverty and lack of access to health care affect not just the disenfranchised. They affect us all, for those who are at greater risk because of these problems are our close neighbors in the sea of pathogens we share. Our society is becoming an increasingly complex organism in which the health of each individual cell— each person—will have impact on the health of the cells around it. No cell is unimportant.

With the "coming of age" of many healing traditions at the same time, we have an unprecedented expansion of options for responding to all these challenges. Their collective wisdom, if harnessed, can guide us in our efforts to create health on an

individual, community, and global basis. Clearly no single tradition has all the answers. A creative integration of the strengths
of all of them will be necessary as we make the transition to
the twenty-first century.

Notes

INTRODUCTION

1. For more information contact: Healthy Cities, 1 Kaiser Plaza, Suite 1930, Oakland, CA 94612, phone (510) 271–2660.

CHAPTER 1
THE CRISIS OF FREEDOM: HOW DO WE CHOOSE?

1. Moscowitz, Jay. 1992. Statement at public meeting of Office of Alternative Medicine Advisory Council, Washington, DC.

2. Reilly, D., M. A. Taylor, N. G. Beattie, et al. 1994. Is evidence for homeopathy reproducible? *The Lancet* (December 10): 1601–6.

323

3. Arnold, J., et al. 1991. Chemopreventive activity of Maharishi Amrit Kalash and related agents in rat tracheal epithelial and human tumor cells. *Proceedings of the American Association for Cancer Research* 32:15–18 (May):128.

4. Brown, M., et al. 1974. The effect of acupuncture on white cell counts. *American Journal of Chinese Medicine* 2(4):383–98.

5. Bush, I. M., et al. 1974. Zinc and the prostate (experimental study). Presentation at the annual meeting of the American Medical Association, Chicago.

6. Champlault, G., et al. 1984. A double-blind trial of an extract of the plant *serenoa repens* in benign prostatic hyperplasia. *British Journal of Clinical Pharmacology* 18:461–62.

7. Kiecolt-Glaser, J., R. Glaser, D. Williger, J. Stout, et al. 1985. Psychosocial enhancement of immunocompetence in a geriatric population. *Health Psychology* 4:25–41.

8. Spiegel D., J. R. Bloom, H. C. Kraemer, and E. Gottheil. 1989. Effects of psychosocial treatment on survival of patients with metastatic breast cancer. *The Lancet* (October 14):888–91.

CHAPTER 2
CHINESE MEDICINE: THE COSMIC SYMPHONY

1. Lytle, C. D. 1993. Monograph. *An overview of acupuncture.* Washington, DC: U.S. Department of Health and Human Services, Public Health Service, Food and Drug Administration, Centers for Devices and Radiological Health.

2. General literature. American Association of Acupuncture and Oriental Medicine, 1994.

3. Helms, J. 1993. Physicians and acupuncture in the 1990s: A Report for the Subcommittee on Labor, Health and Human Services, and Education of the Appropriations Committee. Washington, DC. June 24.

4. As described in Giovanni Maciocia. 1989. *The foundations of Chinese medicine.* New York: Churchill Livingstone.

5. Korngold, E. Personal communication.

6. Beinfield, H. Personal communication.

7. Walker, D. Personal communication.

Notes

8. Connelly, Dianne M. 1979. *Traditional acupuncture: the law of the five elements.* Columbia, MD: The Centre for Traditional Acupuncture: 17.

9. Ibid., 18.

10. Helms, J. Personal communication.

11. Maciocia, 1989, *Foundations of Chinese medicine.*

12. Dharmananda, S. *A Primer on Chinese Herbal Medicine for Medical Doctors.* Available from Portland, OR: Institute for Traditional Medicine.

13. Eisenberg, D. 1985. *Encounters with qi: exploring Chinese medicine.* New York: W. W. Norton and Company.

14. Li, W., and E. J. Lien. 1986. *Fu-zhen* herbs in the treatment of cancer. *Oriental Healing Arts International Bulletin* (January) 11(1):108.

15. Guo, Z. H., et al. 1989. Chinese herb "destagnation" series 1: Combination of radiation with destagnation in the treatment of nasopharyngeal carcinoma (NPC): a prospective randomized trial on 188 cases. *International Journal of Radiation Oncology, Biology, and Physics* 16:297–300.

16. Sun, Y. 1988. The role of traditional Chinese medicine in supportive care of cancer patients. *Recent Results in Cancer Research* 108:327–34.

17. Shiu, W.T.C., et al. 1992. A clinical study of PSP on peripheral blood counts during chemotherapy. *Phytotherapy Research* 6:217–18.

18. Tingliang, J., et al. 1984. Effect of "Liu-Wei-Di-Huang" decoction on prevention and treatment of tumor. *Journal of Traditional Chinese Medicine* 4(1):59–68.

19. Zhang, R., et al. 1990. Medicinal protection with Chinese herb compound against radiation damage. *Aviation, Space, and Environmental Medicine* 61:729–31.

20. Jun, H., et al. 1991. Effects of gynostemma pentaphyllum makino on the immunological function of cancer patients. *Journal of Traditional Chinese Medicine* 11(1):47–52.

21. Li, L., et al. 1992. Observations on the long-term effects of "Yi Qi Yang Yin Decoction" combined with radiotherapy in treatment of nasopharyngeal carcinoma. *Journal of Traditional Chinese Medicine* 12(4):263–66.

22. Ning, C., et al. 1988. Therapeutic effects of *jian pi yi shen* prescription on the toxicity reactions of postoperative chemotherapy in patients with advanced gastric carcinoma. *Journal of Traditional Chinese Medicine* 8(2):113–16.

23. Wang, G. T., et al. 1988. Treatment of operated late gastric carcinoma with prescription of "strengthen the patient's resistance and dispel the

325

invading evil" in combination with chemotherapy: follow-up study of 158 patients and experimental study in animals. Meeting abstract. First Shanghai International Symposium on Gastrointestinal Cancers, November 14–16, Shanghai, China: 244.

24. Boik, J. Summary of research on Chinese herbal medicine and heart disease. Unpublished manuscript available from Laurelhurst Clinic of Oriental Medicine, 2825 S.E. Stark St., Portland, OR 97214, (503) 239–4941.

25. Liao, J., et al. 1988. Pharmacologic effects of codonopsis pilosula-astragalus injection in the treatment of CHD patients. *Journal of Traditional Chinese Medicine* 8(1):1–8.

26. Weng, W., et al. 1984. Therapeutic effect of the crataegus pinnatifida on 46 cases of angina pectoris—a double-blind study. *Journal of Traditional Chinese Medicine* 4(4):293–94.

27. Shan, P., et al. 1984. The beneficial effects of cyclovirobuxine D (CVBD) in coronary heart disease: A double-blind analysis of 110 cases. *Journal of Traditional Chinese Medicine* 4(1):15–19.

28. Shanghai cooperative group. 1984. Therapeutic effect of sodium tanshinone IIA sulfonate in patients with coronary heart disease: A double-blind study. *Journal of Traditional Chinese Medicine* 4(1):20–24.

29. Chen, Y., et al. 1984. Clinical observations on the effects of radix rosae multiflora in reducing blood lipids. *Journal of Traditional Chinese Medicine* 4(4):295–196.

30. Liao, J., et al. Effect of *sheng mai san* on left ventricular performance in coronary heart disease. *Journal of Traditional Chinese Medicine* 2(1):57–62.

31. Guan, M., et al. 1990. Observations on the treatment of coronary heart disease by *kuo guan qu yu ling*. *Journal of Traditional Chinese Medicine* 10(1):49–53.

32. Cooperative group for essential oil of garlic. 1986. The effect of essential oil of garlic on hyperlipemia and platelet aggregation—an analysis of 308 cases. *Journal of Traditional Chinese Medicine* 6(2):117–20.

33. Investigation group on cardiovascular diseases. 1986. Acute myocardial infarction treated with yiqihuoxue mixture: a comparative study of therapeutic effects on 430 patients. *Journal of Traditional Chinese Medicine* 6(3):165–67.

34. Yu, L., et al. 1992. Clinical observations on treatment of 120 cases of coronary heart disease with herba epimedii. *Journal of Traditional Chinese Medicine* 12(1):30–34.

Notes

35. Helms, J. 1995. *Acupuncture energetics: a clinical approach for physicians.* Berkeley, CA: Medical Acupuncture Publishers.

36. Pomeranz, B. 1987. Scientific basis of acupuncture. In *Acupuncture: textbook and atlas,* edited by G. Stux and B. Pomeranz. Heidelberg: Springer-Verlag: 1–34.

37. Pomeranz, B., and G. Stux. 1989. *Scientific bases of acupuncture.* Berlin: Springer-Verlag.

38. Helms, 1995, *Acupuncture energetics.*

39. ter-Riet, G., et al. 1990. Acupuncture and chronic pain: a criteria-based meta-analysis. *Journal of Clinical Epidemiology* 43(11):1191–199.

40. Kleijnen, J., et al. 1991. Acupuncture and asthma: a review of controlled trials. *Thorax* 46(11):799–802.

41. Carlsson, J., et al. 1990. Health status in patients treated with acupuncture or physiotherapy. *Headache* 30(9):593–199.

42. Vincent, C. 1990. The treatment of tension headache by acupuncture: a controlled single case design with time series analysis. *Journal of Psychosomatic Research* 34(5):553–61.

43. Kitade, T., et al. 1990. Studies on the enhanced effect of acupuncture analgesia and acupuncture anesthesia by D-phenylalanine (2nd report)—schedule of administration and clinical effects in low back pain and tooth extraction. *Acupuncture and Electrotherapy Research* 15(2):121–35.

44. Dundee, J. 1990. Belfast experience with P6 acupuncture antiemesis. *Ulster Medical Journal* 59(1):63–70.

45. Dundee, J., et al. 1990. Clinical uses of P6 acupuncture antiemesis. *Acupuncture and Electrotherapy Research* 15(3–4):211–15.

46. Richter, A., et al. 1990. The effect of acupuncture in patients with angina pectoris. *European Heart Journal* 12(2):175–78.

47. Ballegaard, S., et al. 1991. Acupuncture in angina pectoris: does acupuncture have a specific effect? *Journal of Internal Medicine* 229(4):357–62.

48. Ballegaard, S., et al. 1990. Effects of acupuncture in moderate, stable angina pectoris: a controlled study. *Journal of Internal Medicine* 227(1):25–30.

49. Christensen, B., et al. 1992. Acupuncture treatment of severe knee osteoarthritis: a long-term study. *Acta Anesthesiologia Scandinavia* 38(6):518–25.

50. Chen, Y. 1992. Clinical research on treating senile dementia by combining

acupuncture with acupoint injection. *Acupuncture and Electrotherapy Research* 17(2):61–73.

51. Tremeau, M., et al. 1992. Protocol of cervical maturation by acupuncture. *J-Gynecol-Obstet-Biol-Reprod-Paris* 21(4):375–80.

52. Vincent, C. 1989. A controlled trial of the treatment of migraine by acupuncture. *Clinical Journal of Pain* 5(4):305–12.

53. Blom, M., et al. 1992. The effects of acupuncture on salivary flow rates in patients with xerostoma. *Oral Surgery, Oral Medicine, and Oral Pathology* 73(3):293–98.

54. Helms, J. M. 1987. Acupuncture for the management of primary dysmenorrhea. *Obstetrics and Gynecology* 69:51–56.

55. AMA. 1981. Proceedings of the house of delegates. 130th annual convention. Chicago, IL. June 7–11:198–202.

56. Coan, R. M., et al. 1980. The acupuncture treatment of low back pain: a randomized controlled study. *American Journal of Chinese Medicine* 8:181–89.

57. Richardson, P. H., and C. A. Vincent. 1986. Acupuncture for the treatment of pain: a review of evaluative research. *Pain* 24:15–40.

58. Bullock, M. L., et al. 1987. Acupuncture treatment of alcoholic recidivism: a pilot study. *Alcoholism: Clinical Experimental Research* 11:292–95.

59. Bullock, M. L., et al. 1989. Controlled trial of acupuncture on severe recidivist alcoholism. *The Lancet* (June 24):1435–38.

60. Smith, M. Personal communication.

61. L'Association Française d'Acupuncture. 1993. Paris. Unpublished documents.

62. American Association of Medical Acupuncture. 1993. Los Angeles. Unpublished document.

63. Bannerman, R. H. 1979. Acupuncture: the WHO view. *World Health* (English edition): Dec. 24–29.

64. American Foundation of Medical Acupuncture. 1993. Biomedical research on acupuncture: An agenda for the 1990s. Conference summary. Los Angeles.

65. Helms, Joseph. Personal communication.

66. Walker, D. Personal communication.

67. American Association of Acupuncture and Oriental Medicine, information as of January 1995.

CHAPTER 3
AYURVEDA: THE WISDOM OF THE ANCIENTS

1. Frawley, D. 1989. *Ayurvedic healing: a comprehensive guide.* Salt Lake City: Passage Press: 319.

2. Chopra, D. personal communication.

3. Lad, V. 1984. *Ayurveda: the science of self-healing, a practical guide* Santa Fe: Lotus Press: 22.

4. For a more thorough explanation, see Vasant Lad's *Ayurveda: the science of self-healing, a practical guide* (Santa Fe: Lotus Press, 1984) or Deepak Chopra's *Perfect health: the complete mind/body guide* (New York: Harmony Books, 1991).

5. Morton, J. Personal communication.

6. Cravatta, Mary Jo, D.C. Palo Alto, CA. Personal communication.

7. Collinge, W. 1993. *Recovering from chronic fatigue syndrome: a guide to self-empowerment.* New York: Putnam/Perigee.

8. Stuart Rothenberg, M.D. Personal communication.

9. Ibid.

10. Sharma, H., and C. Alexander. Research Review on Maharishi Ayur-Veda: A Comprehensive System of Natural Medicine. Unpublished paper.

11. Frawley, *Ayurvedic healing*, 319.

12. Panchakarma or rejuvenation therapy. Fairfield, IA: Maharishi Ayur-Ved Health Center. Brochure.

13. Sharma, H. 1993. *Freedom from disease: how to control free radicals, a major cause of aging and disease.* Lancaster, MA: Veda Publishing.

14. Sharma, H., A. N. Hanna, E. M. Kauffman, and H. A. Newman. 1992. Inhibition of human low-density lipoprotein oxidation in vitro by Maharishi Ayur-Veda herbal mixtures. *Pharmacology, Biochemistry, and Behavior* 43:1175–82.

15. Sharma, H., C. Dwivedi, B. Satter, K. Gudehithlu, H. Abou-Issa, W. Malarkey, and G. Tejqani. 1990. Antineoplastic properties of Maharishi-

4 against DMBA-induced mammary tumors in rats. *Pharmacology, Biochemistry, and Behavior* 35:767–73.

16. Prasad, K., J. Edwards-Prasad, S. Kentroti, C. Brodie, and A. Vernadakis. 1992. Ayurvedic (science of life) agents induce differentiation in murine neoblastoma cells in culture. *Neuropharmacology* 31:599–607.

17. Engineer, F., H. Sharma, and C. Dwivedi. 1992. Protective effects of M-4 and M-5 on Adriamycin-induced microsomal lipid peroxidation and mortality. *Biochemistry Archives* 8:267–72.

18. Dileepan, N., V. Patel, H. Sharma, and D. Stechschulte. 1990. Priming of splenic lymphocytes after ingestion of an Ayurvedic herbal food supplement: Evidence for an immunomodulatory effect. *Biochemistry Archives* 6:267–74.

19. Arnold, J., B. Wilkinson, E. Korytynski, and V. Steele. 1991. Chemopreventive activity of Maharishi Amrit Kalash and related agents in rat tracheal epithelial and human tumor cells (abstract). *Proceedings of the American Association of Cancer Research* 32:128.

20. Sharma, H., A. Hanna, E. Kauffman, and H. Newman. 1992. Inhibition of human LDL oxidation in vitro by Maharishi Ayur-Veda herbal mixtures. *Pharmacology, Biochemistry, and Behavior* 43:1175–82.

21. Sharma, H., Y. Feng, and R. Panganamala. 1989. Maharishi Amrit Kalash (MAK) prevents human platelet aggregation. *Clin. Ter. Cardiovasc.* 8:227–230.

22. Nader, T. 1987. Maharishi Ayur-Veda Maharasayana: Its safety and effectiveness in animal models of diet-induced tissue damage, in surgically induced brain lesions, and in chemically induced cancer lesions. Paper presented at the Twenty-Eighth Annual Meeting of the Society for Economic Botany, June, University of Illinois, Chicago.

23. Hanna, A., E. Kauffman, H. Newman, and H. Sharma. 1993. Prevention of oxidant stress by Student Rasayana (SR). Paper presented at the International Symposium on Free Radicals in Diagnostic Medicine, October 7–9, Buffalo, New York.

24. Salerno, J., and D. Smith. 1991. The use of sesame oil and other vegetable oils in the inhibition of human colon cancer cell growth in vitro. *Anticancer Research* 11:209–16.

25. Smith, D., and J. Salerno. 1992. Selective growth inhibition of a human malignant melanoma cell line by sesame oil in vitro. *Prostaglandins, Leucotirenes, and Essential Fatty Acids* 46:145–50.

26. Janssen, G. 1989. The application of Maharishi Ayur-Veda in the treat-

ment of ten chronic diseases: a pilot study. *Ned Tijdschr Geneeskd* 5:586–94.

27. Sharma, H., S. Nidich, D. Sands, and E. Smith. 1993. Improvement in cardiovascular (CV) risk factors through Maharishi panchakarma (PK) purification procedure (abstract). *Federation of American Societies of Experimental Biology* 7(4):A801.

28. Schneider, R., K. Cavanaugh, H. Kasture, S. Rothenberg, R. Averbach, D. Robinson, and R. Wallace. 1990. Health promotion with a traditional system of natural health care: Maharishi Ayur-Ved. *Journal of Social Behavior and Personality* 5(3):1–27.

29. Sircar, A. R., R. C. Paper Ahuja, S. M. Natu, B. Roy, and H. Sharma. 1992. Antidiabetic and general effects of Maharishi Ayur-Veda herbal mixture MA-471. Paper presented at the International Convention on Ayur-Veda, All-India Ayurvedic Congress, April, New Delhi, India.

30. Shanbhag, V. 1988. The role of *sankha-bhasma* (an Ayurvedic medicine) in the treatment of acne vulgaris. M.D. thesis, University of Poona. February.

31. Glaser, J. L., D. K. Robinson, and R. K. Wallace. 1991. Improvement in seasonal respiratory allergy with Maharishi Amrit Kalash 5, an Ayurvedic herb immunomodulator. *Proceedings of the American Association of Ayurvedic Medicine* 7(1):6.

32. Sharma, H., S. Hanissian, A. Rattan, S. Stern, and G. Tejwani. 1991. Effect of Maharishi Amrit Kalash on brain opioid receptors and neuropeptides. *Journal of Research and Education in Indian Medicine* 10(1):1–8.

33. Gelderloos, P., H. Ahlstrom, D. Orme-Johnson, D. Robinson, R. Wallace, and J. Glaser. 1990. Influence of a Maharishi Ayur-Vedic herbal preparation on age-related visual discrimination. *International Journal of Psychosomatics* 37:25–29.

34. Stevens, M., J. Campbell, D. Smith, and M. How. 1989. Pilot project: the effects of a sesame oil mouth rinse on the number of oral bacteria colony types. Paper presented at the Eleventh International Symposium on Dental Hygiene, June 28, Ottawa, Canada.

35. Chopra, D. Personal communication.

36. Shanbhag, V. Personal communication.

CHAPTER 4
NATUROPATHIC MEDICINE: THE GREAT CORNUCOPIA

1. Naturopathic and major medical schools: comparative curricula. American Association of Naturopathic Physicians, P.O. Box 20386, Seattle, WA 98102.

2. Lust, B. 1918. *Universal naturopathic directory and buyer's guide*. American Naturopathic Association.

3. Murray, M. Personal communication.

4. Zeff, J. Personal communication.

5. Ullman, D. 1993. *The one minute (or so) healer*. Los Angeles: Jeremy P. Tarcher, Inc.

6. Lust, B. 1918. *Universal directory of naturopathy*. Vol. I. Lust Publications.

7. Hauser, W. E. and J. S. Remington. 1982. Effect of antibiotics on the immune response. *American Journal of Medicine* 72(5):711–16.

8. Murray, M. Personal communication.

9. Pickering, G. Therapeutics: art or science? 1979. *Journal of the American Medical Association* 242:649–53.

10. Nanba, H., et al. 1993. Antitumor activity of orally administered "D-fraction" from maitake mushroom (*grifola frondosa*). *Journal of Naturopathic Medicine* 4(1):9–15.

11. Barrie, S. A., et al. 1987. Comparative absorption of zinc picolinate, zinc citrate, and zinc gluconate in humans. *Agents and Actions* 21(1–2): 223–28.

12. Barrie, S. A., et al. 1987. Effects of garlic oil on platelet aggregation, serum lipids, and blood pressure in humans. *Journal of Orthomolecular Medicine* 2(1):15–21.

13. Blair, D. M., et al. 1991. Intestinal candidiasis, *L. acidophilus* supplementation, and Crooks's questionnaire. *Journal of Naturopathic Medicine* 2(1):33–36.

14. Brown, D., and A. Lange. 1992. A homeopathic proving of *Candida parapsilosis*. *Homeopathic Links* (Spring) 5:21–22.

15. Standish, L., et al. 1992. One year open trial of naturopathic treatment of HIV infection class IV-A in men. *Journal of Naturopathic Medicine* 3(1):42–64.

16. Calabrese, C. Controlled trial of 2% Aescin gel in experimental hematoma. *Planta Medica*. In press.

17. Stretch, E. 1992. Clinical manifestations of HIV in women. *Journal of Naturopathic Medicine* 3:12–19.

18. Hudson, V. 1991. Consecutive case study research of carcinoma in-situ employing eschariotic treatment combined with nutritional therapy. *Journal of Naturopathic Medicine* 2:6–10.

19. Collins, J. C., and P. Mittman. 1990. The physiological effects of colon hydrotherapy. *Journal of Naturopathic Medicine* 1:4–9.

20. Mittman, P. 1990. Double-blind randomized study of urtica dioica in treatment of allergic rhinitis. *Planta Medica* 56:44–47.

21. Standish, L., Naturopathic treatment of HIV infection, 42–64.

22. Kaiser, J. D. 1994. *Immune power: combining holistic and standard medical therapies into the optimal treatment program for HIV*. New York: St. Martin's Press.

23. *The world almanac book of facts, 1993*. New York: Pharos Books: 226.

24. Ornish, D. 1990. Can lifestyle changes reverse coronary heart disease? *The Lancet* 336:129–32. Also *Dr. Dean Ornish's program for reversing heart disease*. 1990. New York: Random House.

25. Hertog, M., E. Feskens, P. Hollman et al. 1993. Dietary antioxidant flavonoids and risk of coronary heart disease: the Zutphen Elderly Study. *The Lancet* (October 25):1007–11.

26. Manson, J., et al. 1993. Research reported at a meeting of the American Heart Association, November 8–12, Atlanta, Georgia.

27. Trentham, D. 1993. Effects of oral administrations of Type II collagen on rheumatoid arthritis. *Science* 261 (5129):1727–29.

28. Giovannucci, E., E. B. Rimm, G. A. Colditz et al. 1993. A prospective study of dietary fat and risk of prostate cancer. *Journal of the National Cancer Institute* 85 (19):1571–79.

29. Goldbohm, R., P. van den Brandt, P. van 't Veer et al. 1994. A prospective cohort study on the relation between meat consumption and the risk of colon cancer. *Cancer Research* 54(3):718–23.

30. *Proceedings of the National Academy of Sciences*. 1994. April 12.

31. Cheney, Paul. 1991. Is CFS caused by a virus? Talk given at the conference on Chronic Fatigue Syndrome: Current Theory and Treatment, Bel-Air, California. May 18.

32. Werbach, M. 1987. *Nutritional influences on illness.* Tarzana, CA: Third Line Press: xi.

33. Werbach, M. 1993. *Nutritional influences on illness.* 2d edition. Tarzana, CA: Third Line Press.

34. Werbach, M. 1991. *Nutritional influences on mental illness.* Tarzana, CA: Third Line Press.

35. AANP. 1993. *Naturopathic medicine: contributions to health care reform.* Submittal prepared in response to a request for information from the Task Force on National Health Reform. AANP, P.O. Box 20386, Seattle, WA 98102.

36. Kelly, M. D. 1991. Hypercholesterolemia: the cost of treatment in perspective. *Southern Medical Journal* 83 (12):1421–125.

37. AANP, 1993, *Naturopathic medicine: contributions to health care reform.*

CHAPTER 5
HOMEOPATHY: THE GRAND PROVOCATEUR

1. Mark Twain. 1890. A majestic literary fossil. *Harper's Magazine.* February:444.

2. Coulter, H. 1977. *Divided legacy.* Vol. 3. Washington, DC: Wehawken.

3. *Proceedings of the House of Delegates of the American Medical Association* 2:50 (1913) and 34:46 (1914) and American Medical Association, *Digest of official actions, 1846–1938*: 146.

4. Riding the coattails of homeopathy. 1985. *FDA Consumer* (March):31.

5. Herbal and homeopathic remedies: finally starting to reach middle America? *OTC News and Market Report.* 1991. (July):223–38.

6. American Institute of Homeopathy, 1585 Glencoe, Denver, CO 80220, (303) 898–5477.

7. Eisenberg, D., et al. 1993. Unconventional medicine in the United States. *The New England Journal of Medicine* 324(4):246–52.

8. Ferley, J. P., et al. 1989. A controlled evaluation of a homeopathic preparation in the treatment of influenza-like syndromes. *British Journal of Clinical Pharmacology* 27:329–35.

Notes

9. American Institute of Homeopathy, 1585 Glencoe, Denver, CO 80220, (303) 898–5477.

10. Gibson, R. G., et al. 1980. Homeopathic therapy in rheumatoid arthritis: evaluation by double-blind clinical therapeutic trial. *British Journal of Clinical Pharmacology* 9:453–59.

11. Jacobs, J., L. Jimenez, S. Gloyd, et al. 1994. Treatment of acute childhood diarrhea with homeopathic medicine: a randomized clinical trial in Nicaragua. *Pediatrics* 93(5):719–25.

12. Ferley, J. P., et al. 1989. A controlled evaluation of a homeopathic preparation in the treatment of influenza-like syndromes. *British Journal of Clinical Pharmacology* 27:329–35.

13. Taylor-Reilly, D., et al. 1986. Is homeopathy a placebo response? Controlled trial of homeopathic potency, with pollen in hay fever as model. *The Lancet* (October 18):881–86.

14. Reilly, D., M.A. Taylor, N.G. Beattie, et al. 1994. Is evidence for homeopathy reproducible? *The Lancet* (December 10):1601–6.

15. Fisher, P., et al. 1990. Effect of homeopathic treatment on fibrositis (primary fibromyalgia). *British Medical Journal* 299:365–66.

16. Kleijnen, J., P. Knipschild, and G. ter Riet. 1991. Clinical trials of homeopathy. *British Medical Journal* 302:316–23.

17. Coulter, H. L. 1973. *Divided Legacy: The Conflict Between Homeopathy and the American Medical Association.* Berkeley: North Atlantic.

18. Bradford, T. L. 1900. *The logic of figures or comparative results of homeopathic and other treatments.* Philadelphia: Boericke and Tafel: 112–46.

CHAPTER 6
MIND/BODY MEDICINE:
THE DANCE OF SOMA AND PSYCHE

1. Dossey, L. 1989. Mind beyond body. In *Healers on healing*, edited by R. Carlson and B. Shield. Los Angeles: Jeremy P. Tarcher, Inc.: 174.

2. Benson, H. Personal communication.

3. Eisenberg, D. M., R. C. Kessler, C. Foster, F. E. Norlock, D. R. Calkins, and T. L. Delbanco. 1993. Unconventional medicine in the United States:

prevalence, costs, and patterns of use. *The New England Journal of Medicine* 328(4):246–52.

4. Benson, H. Personal communication.

5. Engel, G. L. 1977. The need for a new medical model: a challenge for biomedicine. *Science* 196:129–36.

6. Klopfer, B. 1957. Psychological variables in human cancer. *Journal of Projective Techniques* 21:331–40.

7. Benson, H., J. Beary, and M. Carol. 1974. The relaxation response. *Psychiatry* 37:37–46.

8. See Herbert Benson's *The relaxation response* (New York: Avon Books, 1975) and *Beyond the relaxation response* (New York: Berkley Books, 1985).

9. Temoshok, L., and H. Dreher. 1992. *The type C connection: the behavioral links to cancer and your health.* New York: Random House.

10. Olness, K. 1993. Hypnosis: the power of attention. In *Mind/body medicine: How to use your mind for better health*, edited by D. Goleman and J. Gurin. Yonkers, NY: Consumer Reports Books: 278.

11. Medich, C., E. Stuart, J. Deckro, and R. Friedman. 1991. Psychophysiologic control mechanisms in ischemic heart disease: the mind-heart connection. *Journal of Cardiovascular Nursing* 5(4):10–26.

12. Cobb, S., and R. Rose. 1973. Hypertension, peptic ulcer, and diabetes in air traffic controllers. *Journal of the American Medical Association* 224:489–92.

13. Markovitz, J. H., K. A. Matthews, W. B. Kannel, et al. 1993. Psychological predictors of hypertension in the Framingham study: Is there tension in hypertension? *Journal of the American Medical Association* 270:2439–43.

14. Rosenman, R. H., R. J. Brand, C. D. Jenkins, et al. 1975. Coronary heart disease in the Western collaborative group study: final follow-up experience of 8½ years. *Journal of the American Medical Association* 233:872–77.

15. Carney, R., K. Freedland, M. Rich, et al. 1993. Ventricular tachycardia and psychiatric depression in patients with coronary artery disease. *American Journal of Medicine* 95(1):23–28.

16. Morris, P. L., R. G. Robinson, P. Andrzejewski, J. Samuels, and T. R. Price. 1993. Association of depression with 10-year poststroke mortality. *American Journal of Psychiatry* 150:124–29.

17. Berkman, L., L. Leo-Summers, and R. Horwitz. 1992. Emotional support

and survival after myocardial infarction: a prospective, population-based study of the elderly. *Annals of Internal Medicine* 117:1003–9.

18. Kiecolt-Glaser, J., W. Garner, C. Speicher, G. Penn, J. Holliday, and R. Glaser. 1984. Psychosocial modifiers of immunocompetence in medical students. *Psychosomatic Medicine* 46:7–14.

19. Glaser, R., J. Rice, C. Speicher, J. Stout, and J. Kiecolt-Glaser. 1986. Stress depresses interferon production concomitant with a decrease in natural killer cell activity. *Behavioral Neuroscience* 100(5):675–78.

20. Kiecolt-Glaser, J., R. Glaser, E. Strain, et al. 1986. Modulation of cellular immunity in medical students. *Journal of Behavioral Medicine* 9:311–20.

21. Ibid.

22. Glaser, R., J. Rice, C. Speicher, et al. 1985. Stress-related impairments in cellular immunity. *Psychiatry Research* 16:233–39.

23. Kiecolt-Glaser, J., L. Fisher, P. Ogrocki, et al. 1987. Marital quality, marital disruption, and immune function. *Psychosomatic Medicine* 49:13–34.

24. Martin, R. A., and J. P. Dobbin. 1988. Sense of humor, hassles, and immunoglobulin A: evidence for a stress-moderating effect. *International Journal of Psychiatry in Medicine* 18:93–105.

25. Caldwell, C., M. Irwin, and J. Lohr. 1991. Reduced natural killer cell cytotoxicity in depression but not in schizophrenia. *Biological Psychiatry* 30:1131–38.

26. McClelland, D., and C. Kirshnit. 1988. The effect of motivational arousal through films on salivary immunoglobulin. *Psychology and Health* 2:31–52.

27. Temoshok, L. 1985. Biopsychosocial studies on cutaneous malignant melanoma: psychosocial factors associated with prognostic indicators, progression, psychophysiology, and tumor-host response. *Social Science and Medicine* 20:833–40.

28. Temoshok, L., B. Heller, R. Sagebiel, M. Blois, D. Sweet, R. DiClemente, and M. Gold. 1985. The relationship of psychosocial factors to prognostic indicators in cutaneous malignant melanoma. *Journal of Psychosomatic Research* 2:139–53.

29. Buske-Kirschbaum, A., C. Kirschbaum, H. Stierle, H. Lehnert, and D. Hellhammer. 1992. Conditioned increase of natural killer cell activity (NKCA) in humans. *Psychosomatic Medicine* 54:123–32.

30. Benson, H., S. Alexander, and C. Feldman. 1975. Decreased premature

ventricular contractions through the use of the relaxation response in patients with stable ischemic heart disease. *The Lancet* 2:380–82.

31. Leserman J., E. Stuart, M. Mamish, J. Deckro, R. Beckman, R. Friedman, and H. Benson. 1989. Nonpharmacologic intervention for hypertension: long-term follow-up. *Journal of Cardiopulmonary Rehabilitation* 9:316–24.

32. Wells, J., G. Howard, W. Nowlin, and M. Vargas. 1986. Presurgical anxiety and postsurgical pain and adjustment: effects of stress inoculation procedure. *Journal of Consulting and Clinical Psychology* 57:831–53.

33. Mandle, C., A. Domar, D. Harrington, J. Leserman, E. Bozadjian, R. Friedman, and Benson H. 1990. Relaxation response in femoral angiography. *Radiology* 174:737–39.

34. Leserman, J., E. Stuart, M. Mamish, and H. Benson. 1989. The efficacy of the relaxation response in preparing for cardiac surgery. *Behavioral Medicine* (Fall):111–17.

35. Goodale, I., A. Domar, and H. Benson. 1990. Alleviation of premenstrual syndrome symptoms with the relaxation response. *Obstetrics and Gynecology* 75(4):649–55.

36. Kiecolt-Glaser, J., R. Glaser, D. Williger, J. Stout, et al. 1985. Psychosocial enhancement of immunocompetence in a geriatric population. *Health Psychology* 4:25–41.

37. Kiecolt-Glaser, J., R. Glaser, E. Strain, et al. 1986. Modulation of cellular immunity in medical students. *Journal of Behavioral Medicine* 9:311–20.

38. Benson, H. 1977. Systemic hypertension and the relaxation response. *The New England Journal of Medicine* 296:1152–56.

39. Schneider, R. H., F. Staggers, C. N. Alexander, et al. 1991. Stress management in elderly blacks with hypertension: a preliminary report. *Proceedings of the Second International Conference on Race, Ethnicity, and Health: Challenges in Diabetes and Hypertension.* Sponsored by Case Western Reserve University, Salvador Bahia, Brazil.

40. Feher, S. K., L. W. Berger, J. D. Johnson, and J. B. Wilde. 1989. Increasing breast milk production for premature infants with relaxation and imagery. *Advances* 6(2):14–16.

41. Gruber, B., and N. Hall. 1988. Immune system and psychological changes in metastatic cancer patients using relaxation and guided imagery: a pilot study. *Scandinavian Journal of Behavior Therapy* 17:25–45.

42. Imagery influences immune cells. 1991. *Brain/Mind Bulletin* (October) 17(1):1.

43. Collinge, W., and J. Kabbal. Evocative breath therapy and immunoen-hancement: a pilot study. Manuscript submitted for review. The Cancer Support and Education Center, 1035 Pine St., Menlo Park, CA 94025.

44. Blanchard, E., S. Schwartz, J. Suls, M. Geradi, L. Scharff, B. Greene, A. Taylor, C. Berreman, and H. Malamood. 1992. Two controlled evaluations of multicomponent psychological treatment of irritable bowel syndrome. *Behavior Research and Therapy* 30:175–89.

45. Holroyd K., J. Holm, K. Hursey, D. Penzien, G. Cordingly, A. Theofanous, S. Richardson, and S. Tobin. 1988. Recurrent vascular headache: home-based behavioral treatment versus abortive pharmacological treatment. *Journal of Consulting and Clinical Psychology* 56:218–23.

46. Stuart, E., M. Caudill, J. Leserman, C. Dorrington, R. Friedman, and H. Benson. 1987. Nonpharmacologic treatment of hypertension: a multiple-risk-factor approach. *Journal of Cardiovascular Nursing* 1:1–4.

47. Leserman, J., E. Stuart, M. Mamish, J. Deckro, R. Beckman, R. Friedman, and H. Benson. 1989. Nonpharmacologic intervention for hypertension: long-term follow-up. *Journal of Cardiopulmonary Rehabilitation* 9:316–24.

48. Frasure-Smith, N. 1989. Long-term follow-up of ischemic heart disease life stress monitoring program. *Psychosomatic Medicine* 51: 485–512.

49. Ornish, D., S. E. Brown, L. W. Scherwitz, J. H. Billings, W. T. Armstrong, T. A. Ports, S. M. McLanahan, R. L. Kirkeeide, R. J. Brand, and K. L. Gould. 1990. Can life-style changes reverse coronary heart disease? *The Lancet* 336:129–33.

50. Domar, A., M. Seibel, and H. Benson. 1990. The mind/body program for infertility: a new behavioral treatment approach for women with infertility. *Fertility and Sterility* 53(2):246–49.

51. Auerbach, J., T. Oleson, and G. Solomon. 1992. A behavioral medicine intervention as an adjunctive treatment for HIV-related illness. *Psychology and Health* 6:325–34.

52. Collinge, W. 1989. HIV and quality of life: outcomes of a psychosocial intervention program. *Tenth Annual Proceedings*. Society of Behavioral Medicine, San Francisco: 41.

53. Collinge, W. 1988. Psychosocial outcomes of complementary cancer therapy. *Ninth Annual Proceedings*. Society of Behavioral Medicine, Boston: 60–61.

54. This case example is adapted with permission from the *Provider's Manual*, edited by Carol Wells-Federman, M.Ed., R.N., revised edition, October

1992. Boston: Clinical Training in Behavioral Medicine, Mind/Body Medical Institute, New England Deaconess Hospital.

55. Fawzy, I. 1991. A structured psychiatric intervention for cancer patients: changes over time in methods of coping and affective disturbance and in immunological parameters (abstract). *General Hospital Psychiatry* 13:361–62.

56. Fawzy, F., N. Fawzy, C. Hyun, et al. 1993. Malignant melanoma: effects of an early structured psychiatric intervention, coping, and affective state on recurrence and survival 6 years later. *Archives of General Psychiatry* 50:681–89.

57. Spiegel D., J. R. Bloom, H. C. Kraemer, and E. Gottheil. 1989. Effects of psychosocial treatment on survival of patients with metastatic breast cancer. *The Lancet* (October 14):888–91.

58. Devine, E. C., et al. 1992. Effects of psychoeducational care for adult surgical patients: a meta-analysis of 191 studies. *Patient Education and Counseling* 19:129–42.

59. Caudill, M., R. Schnable, P. Zuttermeister, H. Benson, and R. Friedman. 1991. Decreased clinic use by chronic pain patients: response to behavioral medicine intervention. *The Clinical Journal of Pain* 7: 305–10.

60. Orme-Johnson, D. 1987. Medical care utilization and the transcendental meditation program. *Psychosomatic Medicine* 49:493–507.

61. Cunningham, A. J. 1985. The influence of mind on cancer. *Canadian Psychologist* 26:13–19.

62. Simonton, Carl, M.D. Personal communication.

63. Soos, J. 1992. Psychotherapy and counseling with transplant patients. In *Psychiatric aspects of organ transplantation*, edited by J. Craven and G. M. Rodin. New York: Oxford University Press.

64. Soos, J. Personal communication.

CHAPTER 7
OSTEOPATHIC MEDICINE:
STRUCTURE AND FUNCTION AS ONE

1. Quoted in Solit, M. 1962. Study in structural dynamics. *Journal of the American Osteopathic Association* (hereafter cited as JAOA) 62:30–40.

Notes

2. Lane, M. A. 1918. *Dr. Still, founder of osteopathy.* Chicago: The Osteopathic Publishing Company: 21.

3. Korr, I. M. 1987. Quoted in *Osteopathic research: growth and development,* edited by G. W. Northrop. Chicago: American Osteopathic Association: 110.

4. Northrop, G. W. 1966. *Osteopathic medicine: an American reformation.* Chicago: American Osteopathic Association: 22–27.

5. Anderson, W. Personal communication.

6. Burns, L. 1927. The Sunny Slope Laboratory of the A. T. Still Research Institute. *JAOA* (June) 26:856–57.

7. Iwata, J. L., J. J. Rodos, and A. L. Habenicht. 1993. Psychotic and affective disorders compared by osteopathic structural examination (abstract). *JAOA* (September) 93(9):950.

8. Beal, M. C. 1987. Clinical research. In *Osteopathic research*, 86.

9. Krpan, M. F., L. A. Harrington, R. J. Beckman, et al. 1992. Low back pain (LBP) treatment by high velocity low amplitude (HVLA) osteopathic manipulative therapy and effectiveness measured by electromyography (EMG), plasma catecholamines, and beta endorphin (abstract). *JAOA* (October) 92(9):1283.

10. Siehl, D., D. R. Olson, H. E. Ross, and E. E. Rockwood. 1971. Manipulation of the lumbar spine with the patient under general anesthesia: evaluation by electromyography and clinical-neurologic examination of its use for lumbar nerve root compression syndrome. *JAOA* (January) 70:433–40.

11. Hoyt, W. H., F. Shaffer, D. A. Bard, et al. 1979. Osteopathic manipulation in the treatment of muscle contraction headache. *JAOA* (January) 78:322–25.

12. Siehl, D. 1963. Manipulation of the spine under general anesthesia. *JAOA* (June) 62:881–87.

13. Larson, N. J., M. W. Walton, H. H. Hunt, and A. F. Kelso. 1976. A double-blind clinical study of the effects of manipulative treatment of patients with peripheral nerve complaints. *JAOA* (November) 76:209.

14. Larson, N. J., M. W. Walton, and A. F. Kelso. 1980. Effectiveness of manipulative treatment for parastheses with peripheral nerve involvement. *JAOA* (November) 80:216.

15. Knebl, J. A., R. G. Gamber, et al., 1993. Improving functional ability in the elderly by osteopathic manipulative treatment (abstract). *JAOA* (August) 93(8):870.

341

NOTES

ot present proper

16. Stotz, A. D., and R. E. Kappler. 1993. The effects of OMT on the tender points associated with fibromyalgia (abstract). *JAOA* (August) 93(8):866.

17. R. G. Gamber, B. R. Rubin, et al. Treatment of fibromyalgia with osteopathic manipulation and self-learned techniques (abstract). *JAOA* (August) 93(8):870.

18. Lo, K. S., M. L. Kuchera, S. C. Preston, and R. W. Jackson. 1992. Osteopathic manipulative treatment in fibromyalgia syndrome (abstract). *JAOA* (September) 92(9):1177.

19. Noll, D. R., P. N. Bryman, G. P. Gebhardt, and E. V. Masterson. 1992. The efficacy of OMT in the elderly hospitalized with acute pneumonia (abstract). *JAOA* (September) 92(9):1179.

20. Wilson, P. T. 1925. Experimental work in asthma at the Peter Bent Brigham Hospital. *JAOA* (November) 25:212–14.

21. Koch, R. S. 1957. Structural patterns and principles of treatment in the asthmatic patient. *Academy of Applied Osteopathy 1957 Yearbook*. Newark, OH: American Academy of Osteopathy: 71–72.

22. Howell, R. K., T. W. Allan, and R. E. Kappler. 1975. The influence of osteopathic manipulative therapy in the management of patients with chronic obstructive lung disease. *JAOA* (April) 74:757–60.

23. Schmidt, I. C. 1982. Osteopathic manipulative therapy as a primary factor in the management of upper, middle, and pararespiratory infections. *JAOA* (February) 81:382–88.

24. Purse, F. M. 1961. Clinical evaluation of osteopathic manipulative therapy in measles. *JAOA* (December) 61:274–76.

25. Purse, F. M. 1966. Manipulative therapy in upper respiratory infections in children. *JAOA* (May) 65:964–72.

26. Kline, C. A. 1965. Osteopathic manipulative therapy, antibiotics, and supportive therapy in respiratory infections in children: comparative study. *JAOA* (November) 65:278–81.

27. Northrup, T. L. 1961. Manipulative management of hypertension. *JAOA* (August) 60:973–78.

Notes

CHAPTER 8
CHIROPRACTIC: OPENING THE GATES

1. Mootz, R. D. Chiropractic models: current understanding of vertebral subluxation and manipulable spinal lesions. In *Chiropractic family practice: a clinical manual*, edited by J. J. Sweere. Gaithersburg, MD: Aspen Publishers, Inc.: 1992. 2–28.

2. Shekelle, P., et al. 1991. *The appropriateness of spinal manipulation for low-back pain, project overview and literature review.* Santa Monica, VA: Rand Publication R-4025/2-CCR/FCER.

3. Eisenberg, D. M., R. C. Kessler, C. Foster, F. E. Norlock, D. R. Calkins, and T. L. Delbanco. 1993. Unconventional medicine in the United States: prevalence, costs, and patterns of use. *The New England Journal of Medicine* (January 28) 328(4):246–52.

4. Von Kuster, T. 1980. *Chiropractic health care: a national study of cost of education, service, utilization, number of practicing doctors of chiropractic and other key policy issues.* Washington, DC: The Foundation for the Advancement of Chiropractic Tenets and Science.

5. Schafer, R. C., and L. Sportelli. 1987. *Opportunities in chiropractic health care careers.* Lincolnwood, IL: American Chiropractic Association and VGM Career Horizons.

6. Ibid.

7. Oberstein, L. Personal communication.

8. Undated. *Statement on chiropractic standard of care/patient safety.* Clifton, NJ: Federation of Straight Chiropractic Organizations, 1.

9. Meeker, W. Personal communication.

10. Pammer, J. Personal communication.

11. 1992. *Practice guidelines for straight chiropractic: proceedings of the International Straight Chiropractic Consensus Conference.* Chandler, AZ: World Chiropractic Alliance.

12. Meeker, W. Personal communication.

13. Quoted in Krier, B. A. 1992. A lighter touch: Network chiropractors tap gently to release pain in the body and mind. *Los Angeles Times.* April 9.

14. Brennan, P., K. Kokjohn, C. Kaltinger, et al. 1991. Enhanced phagocytic cell respiratory burst induced by spinal manipulation: potential role of substance P. *Journal of Manipulative and Physiological Therapeutics* 14(7):399–408.

NOTES

15. Deyo, R. A. 1983. Conservative therapy for low back pain: distinguishing useful from useless therapy. *Journal of the American Medical Association* 250:1057–62.

16. Carette, S., S. Marcoux, R. Truchon, et al. 1991. A controlled trial of corticosteroid injections into facet joints for chronic low back pain. *The New England Journal of Medicine* (October 3) 325(14):1002–7.

17. Deyo, R. A., N. E. Walsh, D. C. Martin, et al. 1990. A controlled trial of transcutaneous electrical nerve stimulation (TENS) and exercise for chronic low back pain. *The New England Journal of Medicine* (June 7) 322(23):1627–34.

18. Meade, T., et al. 1990. Low back pain of mechanical origin: randomized comparison of chiropractic and outpatient treatment. *British Medical Journal* 300:1431–37.

19. Shekelle, P., A. Adams, M. Chassin, E. Hurwitz, and R. Brook. 1992. Spinal manipulation for low-back pain. *Annals of Internal Medicine* (October 1) 117:7:590–98.

20. Wiesel, S. W. 1984. A study of computer assisted tomography: the indigence of positive CAT scans in an asymptomatic group of patients. *Spine* 9(6):549–51.

21. Jensen, M. C., M. N. Brant-Zawadski, N. Obuchowski, M. T. Modic, D. Malkasian, and J. S. Ross. 1994. Magnetic resonance imaging of the lumbar spine in people without back pain. *New England Journal of Medicine* 331(2):69–73.

22. Quoted in G. Kolata. 1994. Study raises serious doubts about commonly used methods of treating back pain. *New York Times*. July 14: A9.

23. Cimons, M. 1994. Experts push low-tech care for back pain. *Los Angeles Times*. December 9: A1

24. Cherkin, D., and R. McCormack. 1989. Patient evaluation of low back pain care from family physicians and chiropractors. *Western Journal of Medicine* 150:351–55.

25. Deyo, R. A., and A. K. Diehl. 1986. Patient satisfaction with medical care for low back pain. *Spine* 11:28–30.

26. Greenfield, S., H. Anderson, R. Winickoff, et al. 1975. Nurse-protocol management of low back pain—outcomes, patient satisfaction, and efficiency of primary care. *Western Journal of Medicine* 123:350–159.

27. Kane, R. L., D. Olsen, C. Leymaster, et al. 1974. Manipulating the patient, a comparison of the effectiveness of physician and chiropractor care. *The Lancet* 1:1333–36.

28. Overman, S. S., J. W. Larson, D. A. Dickstein, et al. 1988. Physical therapy care for low back pain—monitored program of first contact nonphysician care. *Journal of the American Physical Therapy Association* 68:199–207.

29. Stano, M. 1992. *A comparison of health care costs for chiropractic and medical patients.* Oakland University, School of Business Administration Working Paper 92–01. July, Rochester, MI.

30. Stano, M., J. Ehrhart, and T. Allenburg. 1992. The growing role of chiropractic in health care delivery. *Journal of American Health Policy* (November/December):39–45.

31. Jarvis, K. B., R. B. Phillips, and E. H. Morris. 1991. Cost per case comparison of back injury of chiropractic versus medical management for conditions with identical diagnosis codes. *Journal of Occupational Medicine* (August) 33(8):847–51.

CHAPTER 9
MASSAGE THERAPY AND BODYWORK:
HEALING THROUGH TOUCH

1. Eisenberg, D. M., R. C. Kessler, C. Foster, F. E. Norlock, D. R. Calkins, and T. L. Delbanco. 1993. Unconventional medicine in the United States: prevalence, costs, and patterns of use. *The New England Journal of Medicine* (January 28) 328(4):246–52.

2. Chieppa, J. Personal communication.

3. Upledger, John. Personal communication.

4. Byers, D. 1991. *Better health with foot reflexology.* St. Petersburg, FL: Ingham Publishing, Inc.

5. Fakouri, C., and T. Jones. Relaxation Rx: slow stroke back rub. 1987. *Journal of Gerontological Nursing* 13(2):32–35.

6. Weintraub, M. 1992. Shiatsu, Swedish muscle massage, and trigger point suppression in spinal pain syndrome. *Massage Therapy Journal* (Summer) 31(3):99–109. Also published in *American Journal of Pain Management* (April 1992) 2(2):74–78.

7. Kaard, B., and O. Tostinbo. 1989. Increase of plasma beta endorphins in a connective tissue massage. *General Pharmacology* 20(4):487–89.

8. Zanolla, R., C. Mazeglio, and A. Balzarini. 1984. Evaluation of the results

of three different methods of postmastectomy lymphedema treatment. *Journal of Surgical Oncology* 26:210–13.

9. Yoachim, G. 1983. The effects of two stress management techniques on feelings of well-being in patients with inflammatory bowel disease. *Nursing Papers* 15(47):5–18.

10. Wirth, D. 1990. The effect of Non-contact Therapeutic Touch on the healing rate of full-thickness dermal wounds. *Subtle Energies* 1(1):1–20.

11. Oleson, T., and W. Flocco. 1993. Randomized controlled study of premenstrual symptoms treated with ear, hand, and foot reflexology. *Obstetrics and Gynecology* (December) 82(6):906–110.

12. Field, T., S. Schanberg, F. Scafidi, et al. 1986. Tactile/kinesthetic stimulation effects on preterm neonates. *Pediatrics* (May) 77(5):654–158.

13. Preliminary unpublished data. Touch Research Institute, University of Miami.

14. Field, T., C. Morrow, C. Valdeon, et al. 1992. Massage reduces anxiety in child and adolescent psychiatric patients. *Journal of the American Academy of Child and Adolescent Psychiatry* 31(1):125–31.

15. Weinburg, R. S., and V. V. Hunt. 1979. Effects of structural integration on state-trait anxiety *Journal of Clinical Psychology* (April) 30(2):319–22.

16. Hunt, V. V., and W. W. Massey. 1977. Electromyographic evaluation of Structural Integration. *Psychoenergetic Systems* 2:199–210.

17. Hunt, V. V., W. W. Massey, R. Weinberg, R. Bruyere, and P. M. Hahn. 1977. *A study of structural integration from neuromuscular, energy field, and emotional approaches.* Boulder, CO: Rolf Institute of Structural Integration.

18. Cottingham, J. T., S. W. Porges, and K. Richmond. 1988. Shifts in pelvic inclination angle and parasympathetic tone produced by Rolfing soft tissue manipulation. *Physical Therapy* (September) 68(9):1364–70.

19. Greene, E. Personal communication.

20. Collinge, W. 1988. Psychosocial outcomes of complementary cancer therapy. *Proceedings of the Society of Behavioral Medicine, Ninth Annual Scientific Sessions.* Boston: 60–61.

21. Reprinted with permission from Iona Marsaa Teeguarden, M.A., *The joy of feeling: bodymind acupressure*™ (Tokyo/New York: Japan Publications, 1987), distributed by Putnam, p. 168.

Notes

CHAPTER 10
NEW CHOICES, NEW REALITIES

1. Weil, A. 1988. *Health and Healing*. Boston: Houghton Mifflin, p. 271.

2. Kaiser, J. Personal communication.

3. Many Tibetan prophecies are not available in English and are passed down orally from one teacher to the next. This particular prophecy was gleaned by Barry Bryant, author of *Cancer and Consciousness* (Boston, MA: Sigo Press, 1990), from his extensive studies with a variety of contemporary lamas and teachers of Tibetan medicine.

4. McGinnis, J. M., and W. H. Foege. 1993. Actual causes of death in the United States. *Journal of the American Medical Association* (November 10) 270(18):2207–12.

5. American Cancer Society. 1993. *Cancer facts and figures—1992*: 1.

6. *Statistical abstract of the United States, 1992*. 1993. Washington DC: U.S. Department of Commerce, Bureau of the Census: 82.

7. Altman, Lawrence K. 1992. AIDS scientist fears epidemic of tuberculosis. *San Francisco Chronicle*. February 11:A8.

8. Russell, S. 1991. Battle against deadly hepatitis B. *San Francisco Chronicle*. November 5:A1.

9. Alzheimer's Disease and Related Disorders Association, Inc., 919 North Michigan Avenue, Chicago, IL 60611-1676, 1993.

10. Petersdorf, R., ed. 1983. *Harrison's principles of internal medicine*. 10th edition. New York: McGraw-Hill.

11. Murray, M., and J. Pizzorno. 1990. *Encyclopedia of natural medicine*. London: Macdonald & Co., Ltd.

12. Prevalence of chronic migraine headaches—United States 1980–1989. 1991. *Morbidity and Mortality Weekly Report* (May 14) 40:20.

13. Mermin, L., ed. 1992. *Lyme disease 1991: Patient/physician perspectives*. Lyme Disease Education Project, P.O. Box 55412, Madison, WI 53705.

14. Environmental Protection Agency. 1990. *Toxics in the community: 1988 national and local perspectives*. Washington, DC: USEPA.

15. Kaiser, J. Personal communication.

16. Drug resistant disease on rise, scientists say. 1993. Reuters News Service. May 18.

Index

AAAOM. *See* American Association of Acupuncture and Oriental Medicine

AAMA. *See* American Academy of Medical Acupuncture

AANP. *See* American Association of Naturopathic Physicians

AAO. *See* American Academy of Osteopathy

Abhyanga, 75

ABMP. *See* Associated Bodywork and Massage Professionals

Academy for Guided Imagery, 203

Acne, 63, 83

Acupressure, 4, 31–32, 281, 296–97

Acupuncture, 2, 9, 13–14, 21, 38–41
for anesthesia, 31
for attention deficit disorder, 33
auricular, 24–26
case studies, 17, 20, 28, 39, 42, 45, 48, 53
choosing a practitioner, 49–52, 54
cost-effectiveness, 41

for depression, 33
Five Element, 21–22, 23, 30, 44
illnessess receptive to treatment, 42–43
Japanese, 24
medical, 22–23
organizations, 51–52, 54
physician/nonphysician issue, 50
physiology of effects, 38–40
state regulation, 49–50
for substance abuse, 40–41
treatment procedure, 30–31

Acute remedy (homeopathy), 138

Acyclovir, 176

Adams, James, 235, 238, 243, 251

Adjustments, chiropractic, 245–46, 257

Adriamycin, 79

Agni, 65

AIDS/HIV, 315, 318
and massage therapy, 288, 292
and mind/body medicine, 191
and naturopathy, 115, 118–20, 122

Air, 57, 60

Alcoholism, 34
Alexander, F. M., 280
Alexander Technique, 280, 303–4
Alkaloids, 78
Allen, John J., 33
Allergies, acupuncture for, 42
Allopathic medicine, 5, 7, 134–35
Aloe vera juice, 87
Ama, 65, 75
AMA. *See* American Medical
    Association
American Academy of Medical
    Acupuncture (AAMA), 52, 54
American Academy of Osteopathy
    (AAO), 230
American Association of Acupuncture
    and Oriental Medicine
    (AAAOM), 52
American Association of Naturopathic
    Physicians (AANP), 99–100, 132
American Board of Homeotherapeutics,
    163
American Chiropractic Association,
    263–64
American Chronic Pain Association, 203
American Council of Hypnotist
    Examiners, 203
American Institute of Homeopathy, 134,
    164
American Institute of Vedic Studies, 91
American Massage Therapy Association
    (AMTA), 267, 299, 300–302
American Medical Association (AMA),
    23, 134–35, 207, 234, 258
American Oriental Bodywork Therapy
    Association (AOBTA), 305
American Osteopathic Association
    (AOA), 207, 209, 230
American School of Ayurvedic Sciences,
    91, 94
American Society of Clinical Hypnosis,
    203
AMTA. *See* American Massage Therapy
    Association (AMTA)
Anderson, William, 209, 210, 211
Anesthesia, 31
Animal products, 86, 122
Antibiotics, 2, 107, 140, 165, 317
Antidoting, 140–42, 159

Antioxidant vitamins, 115
Ants, 81
Anxiety, 53, 73
AOA. *See* American Osteopathic
    Association
AOBTA. *See* American Oriental
    Bodywork Therapy Association
Arthritis, 121, 146, 212
Articulatory techniques, 219
Asanas, 74, 81
Associated Bodywork and Massage
    Professionals (ABMP), 305
Association for Network Chiropractic,
    264
Asthma, 9, 140, 141, 153, 184, 243
Asthmatic bronchitis, 225
Atkins, Robert, 128
Attention deficit disorder, 33
Auricular acupuncture, 24–26
Auricular medicine (auriculotherapy), 26
Aurum metallicum, 143
Autogenic training, 179–80
Ayurveda, 3, 5, 7, 55–95, 111, 310
    case studies, 58, 59, 63, 66, 69, 73
    choosing a practitioner, 89–91, 94
    chronotherapy, 76
    costs, 88–89
    daily routine, 92–93
    diagnosis, 70–72
    dietary therapy, 64–65, 66, 67, 69,
        72, 81, 86–87
    Five Elements, 57–58, 60
    and health, 62, 78
    and illness, 62, 64, 65, 66–67, 80–81
    individual constitution, 58, 60–61
    key principles, 58, 60–62, 64–67
    massage, 75, 91
    organizations, 94
    personal results, 87–88
    practitioner-patient relationship, 85
    procedures and techniques, 70–76, 78
    relationship to other forms of
        medicine, 88
    scientific support, 77–84
        human studies, 80–84
        laboratory studies, 79–80
        strengths and limitations, 84–85
    training for, 89–90
        programs, 90–91, 94

350

variations within tradition, 67–68, 70
vital energy, 57
Ayurveda Holistic Center of New York, 94
Ayurvedic Institute, 90–91

Back pain
chiropractic for, 223, 232, 250–54, 255
massage for, 269
osteopathy for, 223
Bacon, Francis, 1
Balance disorders, 33
Bastyr University of Natural Health Sciences, 91, 97, 115, 129
Beal, Myron, 223
Beck, Bridget, 291
Beinfeld, Harriet, 16, 17, 20, 25, 28, 39
Benson, Herbert, 168, 169, 174, 177, 201
Biochemical approach, 109
Biofeedback, 182–83, 184, 190
Biofeedback Certification Institute of America, 203
Bladder, 101, 131, 165
Blood circulation, 211, 268, 270
Bodily system enhancement, 270
Bodymind Acupressure™, 282
Bodywork, 266–306, 311
case studies, 292, 301
choosing a practitioner, 302–6
costs, 298–99
education for, 268
key principles, 268, 270–71
organizations, 303–6
personal results, 297–98
practitioner-patient relationship, 295, 297
relationship to other forms of medicine, 298
research, 293
scientific support, 287–93
strengths and limitations, 293–95
varieties and techniques, 271–78, 280–83, 285–87
Botanical medicine, 110–11
Bowel movements, 66, 108
Brain, 171
Breast cancer, 193

Breast-feeding, 157, 189
Breath therapy, 180, 189–90
Broccoli, 122
Brooks, Sister Anne, 212
Burk, Thomas, 288
Burns, Louisa, 221–22

Canadian College of Naturopathic Medicine, 97, 129
Cancer
breast, 193
and Chinese herbs, 34–36
colon, 122
herbal rasayanas for, 79
and homeopathy, 156–57
and macrobiotic diet, 115
and massage therapy, 294–95
and mind/body medicine, 171, 175, 181, 184, 186–87, 191, 193, 195, 196
and naturopathy, 115, 126
prostate, 1, 121–22
Cancer Support and Education Center, 201
Carlston, Michael, 139, 141–42, 144, 156
Carroll, Karen, 170
CCE. See Council on Chiropractic Education
Center for Attitudinal Healing, 203
Center for Mind/Body Medicine, 56, 68, 91, 202–3
Cesarean section, 125
Champa, 63
Chemotherapy, 79–80, 115
Chest pain, 45
Chi, 2, 3, 15–16, 32, 281
and acupuncture, 21–22, 32, 40, 48
and diagnosis, 27
and modern health problems, 18–19
and treatment of illness, 18
Chicken cartilage, 121
Chieppa, Joanna, 271, 304
Chi kung, 3, 32, 33
Children
diarrhea, 152
and drugs, 157
ear infections, 123, 140, 156, 248–49
homeopathy for, 152, 156

351

Children (*cont.*)
  measles, 226
  respiratory infections, 226
Chinese herbs, 2, 21, 29–30, 34–37, 39
Chinese medicine, 2, 5, 7, 13–54, 111,
    310
  case studies, 17, 20, 25, 28, 35, 39,
    42, 45, 48
  costs, 47
  diagnosis, 26–28
  eclectic, 26
  ethnic traditional, 23
  insurance coverage, 47
  key principles, 14–19
  meaning of symptoms, 16, 18, 26
  and modern health problems, 18–19
  personal results, 45–46
  practitioner-patient relationship, 44
  relationship to other forms of
    medicine, 46
  scientific support, 32–41
  strengths and limitations, 41–43
  traditional, 20–21, 27
  treatment of illness, 18, 29–32
  varieties of, 19–26
  See also Acupuncture
Chiropractic, 3, 232–65, 311
  before treatment, 244–45
  case studies, 235, 238, 243, 251, 254,
    256–57, 259, 262, 265
  choosing a practitioner, 261–63
  costs, 254–55, 260–61
  education, 235–36
  follow-up care, 247
  history of, 233–34
  key principles, 236–40
  manipulation, 233, 244, 245–46, 249,
    250–52, 257, 259
  network, 244, 246
  organizations, 263–64
  personal results, 258
  practitioner-patient relationship, 257
  procedures and techniques, 244–47
  relationship to other forms of
    medicine, 258–60
  scientific support, 247–55
  "straights" and "mixers," 241–42,
    263
  strengths and limitations, 255, 257

subluxation, 237–39, 240, 242–44,
    263
  therapies, 245–47
  treatment for low back pain, 250–54,
    255
  patient satisfaction, 253
  variations within tradition, 240–44
Chopra, Deepak, 56, 67, 89, 91, 202–3
Chronic fatigue syndrome, 67, 116, 122,
    160, 176
Chronic obstructive lung disease, 225
Chronic remedy (homeopathy), 138
Chronotherapy, 76
Chyawanprash, 79
Circulatory system, 171
Classical acupuncture. *See* Acupuncture,
    Five Element
Classical homeopathy, 144–45, 148–49,
    151–52
Coffee, 141
College of Maharishi Ayur-Ved, 68, 91
Colon, 122
Combination homeopathy, 147
Common cold, 102–3
Commonweal Cancer Help Program,
    201
Condiments, 87
Connelly, Dianne, 22
Consciousness, 68, 70
Consortium for Chiropractic Research,
    247–48
Constitutional remedy (homeopathy),
    138, 144, 157
Convulsions, 165
Copeland, Royal, 135
Coping styles, 174–75
Coronary heart disease. *See* Heart
    disease
Council for Homeopathic Certification,
    160, 163
Council on Chiropractic Education
    (CCE), 235
Council on Homeopathic Education,
    162, 166
Council on Naturopathic Medical
    Education, 97, 132
Cranial Academy, 230–31
Cranial manipulation, 219–21, 246
Craniosacral manipulation, 259, 262

CranioSacral Therapy™, 285–86
Cravatta, Mary Jo, 64, 69, 73
Crawford, Helen, 184
Cunningham, Alastair, 195

Dairy, 87
Deep tissue massage, 274
DeGood, Douglas, 288
DeJarnette, Major B., 221, 246
Dental drilling, 141
Depression, 33, 143, 157, 185, 186, 291
Detoxification, 105–6
Devine, Elizabeth, 194
Diabetes, 82–83, 112, 184
Diarrhea, 152
Diet
   Ayurvedic, 64–65, 66, 67, 69, 72, 81,
      86–87
   hypoallergenic, 116
   macrobiotic, 115
   naturopathic, 106, 110, 115, 116,
      119, 120, 122–24, 126
Docere (doctor as teacher), 101–2
Dong chong xia cao worm, 51
Dosha, 3, 60, 62, 64–65, 71, 72, 75
Drug addiction
   acupuncture for, 24, 40–41
   Ayurveda for, 78
Drugs
   children's use of, 157
   over the counter, 135
   overuse of, 135–36
   resistance to, 317
Dubin, Robert, 246, 257, 259
Duhl, Leonard, 320

Ear
   auricular acupuncture, 24–26
   infections, 123, 140, 156, 248–49
Earache, 124
Earth, 57, 61
Eastern thought, 5
EBT. *See* Evocative breath therapy
Eczema, 243
Eddy, David, 7
Eight Principles, 21, 23
Eisenberg, David, 168, 232
Electrical stimulation, 245
Electrodermal (EDR) biofeedback, 182

Electromyographic (EMG) biofeedback,
   182
Energetic therapies, 308, 310–11
Energy, 271
   See also Chi
Engel, George, 169–70
Environmental medicine, 111
Epstein, Donald, 244, 246
Erskine, Yusuf, 218, 219
Esalen massage, 273–74
Ether, 57, 60
Evocative breath therapy (EBT), 180,
   189–90
Exercise, 3

Family history, 5
FDA. *See* Food and Drug
   Administration
Feces, 65
Feldenkrais, Moshe, 278
Feldenkrais Method, 278, 280, 303
Fever, 165
Fibromyalgia, 153, 224–25
Field, David, 42, 108, 112
Field, Tiffany, 290
Fight-or-flight reaction. *See* Stress
   response
Finger pulse biofeedback, 182
Fire, 57, 61
Fitzgerald, William, 286
Five Elements, 58, 60
Flavonoids, 121
Food. *See* Diet
Food and Drug Administration (FDA),
   135
Foster, James, 97
Foundation for Chiropractic Education
   and Research, 248
Foundation for Homeopathic Education
   and Research, 166
Frawley, David, 55, 68, 91
Freedom from Disease (Sharma), 79
Fruits, 86, 120
Fu-zhen herbs, 34–35

Gallstones, 59
Gardener, Gail, 301
Ginnandes, Carol, 184
Gold, 143

Grains, 86
Gray, H., 13
Greene, Elliot, 267, 269, 275, 279, 284, 294

Haas, Elson, 124, 128, 316
Hahnemann, Samuel, 136, 137, 145
Hain, Timothy, 33
Halper, James, 184
Han Dynasty, 14
Hatha yoga, 78
Headache, 155, 223–24, 284
    See also Migraine headaches
Healing and the Mind (TV series), 31, 168
Heart attack, 121, 185, 190
Heart disease
    and Chinese herbs, 36–37
    and homeopathy, 157
    and mind/body connection, 175, 185, 190–91
    and naturopathy, 120–21
Heller, Joseph, 277
Hellerwork, 277, 298, 303
Helms, Joseph, 23, 38, 43, 46
Herbal approach, 307–8, 310–11
Herbal medicine. See Botanical medicine
Herbs
    Ayurvedic, 3, 9, 70, 72–74, 79, 81, 83, 90
    Chinese, 2, 21, 29–30, 34–37, 39
Herniated disc, 224, 252, 256–57
Heroin addiction, 78
Herpes, 156
Herrick, Nancy, 139, 142, 156
High velocity-low amplitude thrust techniques, 219
Hippocrates, 100, 135, 266
HIV. See AIDS/HIV
Holism, 210, 237
Holland, Carlisle, 208, 214, 216, 217, 219, 220, 227
Holographic imprint, 137
Homeopathic Academy of Naturopathic Physicians, 132, 164
Homeopathic Educational Services, 166
Homeopathy, 3, 110, 134–66, 310
    antidoting, 140–42, 159

case studies, 140, 143, 146, 155, 157, 161, 165
choosing a practitioner, 160–62
classical, 144–45, 148–49, 151–52
costs, 160
education and training, 162–64
healing process, 142–43
interview process, 148
key principles, 135–44
law of similars, 135–36, 145
nonclassical, 146–47, 149–50
organizations, 164
    certifying, 163–64
personal results, 158–59
practitioner-patient relationship, 158
procedures and techniques, 148–50
relationship to other forms of medicine, 159
remedies, 136–37, 138, 142–50, 157
role of symptoms, 138–40, 142, 144, 148, 157
scientific support, 150–51
    controlled clinical trials, 151–55
strengths and limitations, 155–58
variations within tradition, 144–47
vital force, 137, 139, 144
Homeostasis, 211, 213
Hydrotherapy, 96, 110, 112, 119, 123
Hypertension, 190, 192, 211, 226
Hypnosis, 180, 182, 184
Hypnotherapy, 3

Ice, 245
Imagery, 3, 179, 181, 184, 189, 196, 198
Immune system, 67, 107, 171, 179, 184, 185–87, 248–49
India, 56, 78, 89
Infertility, 191
Inflammation, 102
Inflammatory bowel disease, 289
Innate Intelligence, 233–34, 236, 237, 244
Insight Meditation Society, 201
Insight Meditation West, 201
Insurance
    for Chinese medicine, 47
    for naturopathy, 129
Integrative medicine, 313–18

Intelligence, 80
International Chiropractic Association, 263
International Foundation for Homeopathy (IFH), 165–66
Isopathy, 147

Jacobs, Jennifer, 152
Japanese acupuncture, 24
Jasnoski, Mary, 184
Jing energy, 39
Jin Shin Do®, 282, 305
Jin Shin Jyutsu, 281–82, 304, 305
Joint mobilization, 218
Justice, Blair, 184

Kabat-Zinn, Jon, 178, 201
Kaiser, Jon, 118, 128, 315, 318
Kapha, 3, 60, 61, 62, 69, 71
Kenner, Dan, 45, 48, 53
Kidney disease, 202
Klopfer, Bruno, 172
Kneipp, Sebastian, 96
Korngold, Efrem, 16
Krag, Martin, 248
Krebiozen, 172
Krieger, Dolores, 282–83
Kunz, Dora, 283
Kushi, Lawrence, 115

Laboratory testing, 149
Lad, Vasant, 57, 64, 68, 90
Lane, Michael, 205
Law of similars, 135–36
Legumes, 86
Life span, 84
Lifestyle, 175, 240
Lillard, Harvey, 233
Ling, Per Henrik, 273
Low back pain, 223, 250–54, 255
Lungs, 225
Lust, Benedict, 96–97, 98–99, 105–6
Lymphatic fluid movement, 270
Lymphatic pump, 218
Lymphedema, 289

Macrobiotic diet, 115
Maharishi Amrit Kalash (MAK-4/5), 79, 83–84

Maharishi Ayur-Ved, 68, 70, 74, 76, 77, 81
Maharishi Ayur-Veda Maharasayana, 80
Maharishi Ayur-Ved Medical Association, 94
Maharishi Ayur-Ved Products International, 94, 203
Maharishi International University, 68, 91
Maharishi Mahesh Yogi, 68
MAK-4/MAK-5. *See* Maharishi Amrit Kalash
Malignant melanoma, 186, 191, 193
Manipulation
    cranial, 219–21, 246
    craniosacral, 259, 262
    See also Chiropractic, manipulation; Osteopathy, manipulation
Manson, JoAnn, 121
Manual lymph drainage massage, 276
Manyam, Bala V., 78
Marma points, 75, 81
Massage, 2, 3, 4, 266–306, 311
    Ayurvedic, 75, 91
    case studies, 269, 275, 279, 284, 296–97, 304
    choosing a practitioner, 299–302
    contemporary Western, 273–76
    costs, 298–99
    education for, 268
    in elderly, 287, 289
    energetic methods (nonoriental), 282–83, 285
    key principles, 268, 270–71
    miscellaneous approaches, 285–87
    Oriental methods, 281–82
    personal results, 297–98
    practitioner-patient relationship, 295, 297
    relationship to other forms of medicine, 298
    scientific support, 287–93
    strengths and limitations, 293–95
    structural/functional/movement integration, 276–78, 280
    traditional European, 272–73
    varieties and techniques, 271–78, 280–83, 285–87
    See also Acupressure

355

McGrady, Angele, 184
Measles, 226
Meat, 122
Medications. *See* Drugs
Medich, Cynthia, 183
Medicine
  benefits of diversity, 10–11
  choosing form of, 4–6
    economic considerations, 6
    philosophical/religious
      considerations, 5
    proximity as factor, 6
    relationship with practitioner, 5
    and scientific support, 6
  integrative, 313–14, 316–18
  quest for "scientific," 6–9
  research in, 9–10
  traditions in, 8, 11–12
  treatment outcomes, 8
  See also specific forms, e.g., Chinese
    medicine
Meditation, 67, 70, 74–75, 177–78,
  188–89
Meeker, William, 239, 257, 260
Mental imagery. *See* Imagery
Mentastics, 278
Meridians, 16, 27, 31, 32, 281
Metanalysis, 153–54
Migraine headaches, 141, 143, 155, 160
Mind/body connection, 171–72, 183,
  185–87, 271
Mind/Body Medical Institute, 168, 201
Mind/body medicine, 9, 167–204, 310
  case studies, 170, 176, 181, 192, 196,
    198, 202
  choosing a practitioner, 200–201
  coping styles, 174–75
  costs, 194, 199–200
  key principles, 169–75
  and lifestyle, 175
  multistrategy group programs,
    190–91, 193
  organizations and resources, 201–4
  personal results, 198–99
  practitioner-patient relationship, 197
  procedures and techniques, 177–80,
    182–83, 187–90
  relationship to other forms of
    medicine, 199

relaxation response, 168, 174,
  177–79, 187–88
  scientific support, 183–94
  strengths and limitations, 195–97
  stress response, 173, 185–86
  variations of, 176–77
Mindfulness, 178
Mitral valve prolapse, 208
Mootz, Robert, 232
Morrison, Roger, 141, 149, 156, 160
Morton, Janhavi, 64
Moxibustion, 31
Moyers, Bill, 31, 168
Murray, Michael, 99, 114, 124, 128
Muscle energy manipulation, 218–19
Musculoskeletal system, 206, 210,
  223–25, 239, 270
Myofascial release, 219
Myofibrositis, 224

NACSCAOM. *See* National
  Accreditation Commission for
  Schools and Colleges of
  Acupuncture and Oriental
  Medicine
NASH. *See* North American Society of
  Homeopaths
Nasya, 58
National Accreditation Commission for
  Schools and Colleges of
  Acupuncture and Oriental
  Medicine (NACSCAOM), 52
National Center for Homeopathy
  (NCH), 164
National College of Chiropractic, 249
National College of Naturopathic
  Medicine, 97, 126, 129
National Commission for Certification
  of Acupuncturists (NCAA),
  51–52
National Institutes of Health. *See* Office
  of Alternative Medicine (NIH)
Natural killer (NK) cells, 186, 188
Naturopathy, 2, 9, 96–133, 310, 313
  case studies, 101, 105, 108, 112, 116,
    119, 120, 123, 124, 127, 131
  choosing a practitioner, 129–32
  costs, 124–25, 129
  detoxification, 105–6

dietary therapy, 106, 110, 116, 119, 120, 122–24, 126
education and training for, 97–98, 129–30
healing and symptoms, 102–4
history of, 96–97
key principles, 98–107
licensing, 130–31
and modern illness, 106–7
organizations, 132
personal results, 127–28
practitioner-patient relationship, 126–27
procedures and techniques, 113–14
relationship to other forms of medicine, 128
scientific support, 114, 116–25
mainstream, 118–24
recent studies, 117–18
strengths and limitations, 125–26
treatment modalities, 109–13
unifying philosophy, 99–102
varieties of, 107–13
NCAA. *See* National Commission for Certification of Acupuncturists
NCH. *See* National Center for Homeopathy
Nei Jing, The, 14
Nervous system, 171, 234, 240
Neuromuscular massage, 274
Newton, Patricia, 184
NIH. *See* Office of Alternative Medicine (NIH)
NK cells. *See* Natural killer (NK) cells
Nogier, Paul, 25
Nonclassical homeopathy, 146–47, 149–50
North American Society of Homeopaths (NASH), 163
Nutritional approach, 307–8, 310–11
Nuts, 87

Oberstein, Larry, 238
Obsessive compulsive disorder, 77
Obstetrics, naturopathic, 111, 125
Office of Alternative Medicine (NIH), 6, 33, 77, 115, 151, 168, 184, 248, 288
Oils, 87

Olson, Melodie, 288
Ornish, Dean, 120, 125, 128, 316
Ortho-Binomy, 280
Osler, W., 13
Osteochondrosis, 265
Osteopathy, 4, 205–31, 311
case studies, 208, 212–13, 217, 220
choosing a practitioner, 230
costs, 229–30
current status, 207, 209
diagnosis, 216
education and training, 209–10
emphasis on structure and function, 210–11
history of, 205–7
as integrative medicine, 215–16
key principles, 210–11, 213–14
manipulation in, 226–27
organizations, 230–31
personal results, 228–29
practitioner-patient relationship, 228
relationship to other forms of medicine, 229
scientific support, 221–26
specializations, 215
strengths and limitations, 226–28
treatment, 217–21
variations within tradition, 214–16
OTC drugs. *See* Over-the-counter (OTC) drugs
Otitis media. *See* Ear, infections
Over-the-counter (OTC) drugs, 135

Pain
acupuncture for, 38, 40, 45
massage therapy for, 289, 304
mind/body techniques for, 170, 184, 194
See also Back pain
Palmer, B. J., 234, 263
Palmer, D. D., 233, 236, 237
Palpation, 285
Pammer, John, 239, 255
Panchakarma, 59, 75–76, 80, 81, 82, 89, 91
Panic attacks, 73
Parkinson's disease, 78
Pauls, Arthur Lincoln, 280
Peripheral nerves, 224

Physical medicine, 110
Physiotherapy, 245
Pitta, 3, 59, 60, 61, 62, 63, 66, 69, 71, 72, 86
Pizzicilli, 76
Placebos, 152–53, 167
PMS. See Premenstrual syndrome
Pneumonia, 225
Polarity therapy, 283, 285
Positioning techniques, 219
Potentization, 136
Prakriti, 60, 62, 71
Prana, 57, 73
Pranayama, 57, 73, 74
Prasad, Kedarn, 115
Pregnancy, 157
Premenstrual syndrome (PMS), 66, 188, 290
Prevention, 84, 101, 144, 214
Primum no nocere (first do no harm), 100–101
Progressive relaxation, 178–79
Prostate, 1–4, 9, 35, 121–22
Prostate specific antigen test, 1
Proving (remedy testing method), 150
Psychological medicine, 111
Psycho-neuro-immunology, 171
Psychosocial morbidity, 197
Psychotherapy, 3
Psychotic patients, 222
Pulse diagnosis, 27, 45–46, 71, 90

Qi. See Chi
Qi gong. See Chi kung

Radiation therapy, 115
Rasayanas, 72–75, 79, 83
Reflexology, 286, 290, 306
Reflex sympathetic dystrophy, 33
Reflux esophagitis, 127
Reiki, 285
Relaxation response, 3, 168, 174, 177–79, 187–88
Research, 9–10, 293
    bodywork, 293
Respiratory infections, 226
Restimulation, 213–14

Retinitis pigmentosa, 119
Retzlaff, Ernest, 285
Rheumatoid arthritis, 121, 146, 212
Rib raising. See Lymphatic pump
Rishis, 55
Rolf, Ida, 276
Rolfing, 4, 276–77, 291, 293, 298
Rolf Institute of Structural Integration, 276, 303
Rondberg, Terry, 242
Rosen, Marion, 277
Rosen Method, 277–78, 295, 301, 303
Rothenberg, Stuart, 68, 71

Salivary immunoglobulin A (S-IgA), 186, 189–90
Salk, Jonas, 318
Saw palmetto, 9
Scafidi, Frank, 288
Scientific methods, 8–9
Seeds, 87
Segmental dysfunction, 237
Self-knowledge, 55
Sesame oil, 75, 80, 84
Sex, 2, 3
Shaffer, Howard, 78
Shanbhag, Vivek, 59, 63, 76, 90, 92, 94
Shankha bhasma, 63, 83
Shannahoff-Khalsa, David, 78–79
Sharma, Hari, 79
Shen disturbances, 53
Sherman, Richard, 184
Shiatsu, 31–32, 281
Shirodhara, 76
Shoulder, 224
Simon, David, 78
Simonton, Carl, 198
Single-remedy homeopathy, 145
Skin, 25, 28, 119
Smith, Michael, 40
Sodhi, Virender, 68, 91
Somatic approach, 307, 310–11
Somatic dysfunction, 214
Soos, John, 202
Southwest College of Naturopathic Medicine and Health Sciences, 97, 130
Spine, 233, 246, 249, 250–52, 253, 257, 260, 289

Spontaneous Healing (Weil), 318
Sports massage, 274–75
Standish, Leanna, 118
Still, Andrew Taylor, 205–6
Stone, Randolph, 283
Stress, 3, 271
  acupuncture for, 48
  and Ayurveda, 66
Stress Reduction Clinic, University of
    Massachusetts Medical Center,
    201
Stress response, 173, 185–86
Student Rasayana, 80
Subluxation, 237–39, 240, 242–44, 263
Substance abuse. See Drug addiction
Substance P, 249
Sulforaphane, 122
Sun Salute, 74
Surgery, 81, 111, 188, 198, 252
Susruta Samhita, 81
Sutherland, William, 219–21, 231, 246,
    285
Sweat, 65
Swedish/Esalen massage, 273–74
Swedish massage, 272–73
Sweeteners, 87

Tai chi, 33
Taxol, 9
Taylor, Charles and George, 272
TCM. See Chinese medicine, traditional
Teeguarden, Iona Marsaa, 282
Temoshok, Lydia, 175, 186
Tension release, 270
Therapeutic Touch, 282–83, 288,
    289–90, 305
Thermal biofeedback, 182
Thoracic pump. See Lymphatic pump
TM. See Transcendental meditation
Tolle causam (identify and treat the
    cause), 101
Tope, Denise Matt, 288
Total Health catalog, 94
Touch Research Institute (University of
    Miami), 290–93
Toxemia, 106
Toxin release, 270
Traction, 245–46

Trager, Milton, 278
Trager approach, 278, 303
Transcendental meditation (TM), 68,
    70, 74, 174, 188–89, 194
Treadway, David, 94
Tridosha, 60, 64, 71

Ullman, Dana, 137, 145, 154, 164
Ultrasound, 245
Upledger, John, 212, 221, 285,
    286
Upledger Institute, 305–6
Urethritis, 35
Urine, 65

Vata, 3, 59, 60–61, 62, 64, 66–67, 71,
    72, 73, 86
Vedas, 55
Vedic astrology, 55
Vedic sciences, 55
Vedic Sciences Institute, 94
Vegetables, 86
Vertebra, 237
Vikriti, 65, 71
Vis medicatrix naturae (healing power
    of nature), 100, 107
Vital force, 137, 139, 144
Vitalistic approach (naturopathy),
    107–9
Vitalistic perspective, 309, 312
Vitalistic principle (chiropractic),
    236–37
Vitamins, 122
  antioxidant, 115
  and heart attack, 121

Walker, David, 19, 21, 43
Waste materials, bodily, 65
Water, 57, 61
Weil, Andrew, 128, 307, 318
Wellness Community, 203
Werbach, Melvyn, 122–23, 128
Wilk, Chester, 234
World Chiropractic Alliance,
    264
Worsley, J. R., 21
Wound healing, 289–90
Wu, Wen-Hsien, 33

Yellow Emperor's Classic of Internal Medicine, The, 14
Yin and yang, 15, 21
Yoga, 55, 74, 78, 81
YogAyu, 94

Zeff, Jared, 100, 102, 106, 119, 123, 126, 131
Zero balancing, 286–87, 306
Zinc, 9
Zone therapy, 286
Zovirax, 156

About the Author

William Collinge, Ph.D., is on the Board of Advisors of the American Holistic Health Association. He is clinical supervisor at the Cancer Support and Education Center, Menlo Park, CA, which conducts an intensive mind/body program for people with illness; and research director at the Flowing River Institute, San Francisco, which explores innovations in integrative medicine. His special interests are in meditation, breath therapy, and cultivating vital energy.

He is also the author of *Recovering from Chronic Fatigue Syndrome: A Guide to Self-Empowerment* (Putnam/Perigee, 1993).

He received an M.P.H. and Ph.D. from the University of California, Berkeley, where he was a Murphy Fellow of the American Cancer Society. A licensed psychotherapist, he received clinical training in behavioral medicine at Harvard's Mind/Body Medical Institute.

Dr. Collinge has produced audiotape programs applying the principles of mind/body medicine to cancer, chronic fatigue syndrome, HIV, heart disease, hypertension, gastrointestinal disorders, preparation for and recovery from surgery, stress reduction, and health enhancement. For information, contact: William Collinge, Ph.D., P.O. Box 2002, Sebastopol, CA 95473.